Odyssey
of a
Physician-Scientist

John Ross, Jr. M.D.
Distinguished Professor of Medicine Emeritus
University of California San Diego School of Medicine

Copyright © 2014 John Ross, Jr. M.D.
All rights reserved.
ISBN: 1494786729
ISBN-13: 9781494786724
Library of Congress Control Number: 2014900068
CreateSpace Independent Publishing Platform
North Charleston, South Carolina

This book is dedicated to Eugene Braunwald, MD, my mentor and colleague and Lola Romanucci-Ross, PhD, the light of my life.

CHAPTER 1
PROLOGUE TO A CAREER

Bronxville, a well-to-do, well-segregated community in Westchester County, was my hometown. It was (still is) one square mile, filled with large houses, attractive clubs, and churches, and what was considered an outstanding public (practically private) school. Among my vivid memories of the 1930s, in this town filled with bank presidents, CEOs, and inherited money, is a dinner table conversation at my parents' house concerned with keeping Bronxville closed to blacks and Jews. I remember that the outspoken wife of a prominent physician in the community suddenly announced from her chair, "I will not die in peace until I have a black and a Jew sitting at my right and my left at a dinner table such as this." The stunned silence that followed her proclamation spoke for itself. And the effect on me? That event began my own awareness and questioning and led to my decision never to settle in Bronxville.

Immediate Predecessors

My father, John Ross (no middle name), was born on his father's farm in East Tennessee in a region adjacent to the Great

Smoky Mountains. His mother, Tennessee ("Tenny") Armstrong Ross, died in childbirth when he and his two brothers were very young,. The boys were then raised by a stepmother who had her own (preferred) children by my father's father, George Washington Ross. All three brothers from the initial family worked their way through college. The youngest, Lanty, became superintendent of schools for the county. My father left for college with a trunk filled with apples because he had little else to take: the apples reduced his food bill in the winter, and he supported himself by teaching Latin. Eventually, he followed his older brother, Samuel T. Ross, to medical school at Vanderbilt University in Nashville, Tennessee (classes of 1915 and 1920, respectively). Dr. Sam Ross became a prominent surgeon in Nashville, and my father, while interning at Vanderbilt University Hospital, met and married my mother, Janet Moulder. In the early 1920s, they moved to New York City, where my father became established as one of the early ear, nose, and throat specialists (otorhinolaryngology), initially working with a more senior specialist. As a boy, I often accompanied my father as he drove to his office at Six East Seventieth Street, just across the street from the Frick Museum (which I often visited because of its art collection). I watched him work at his office, as well as at the Saint Luke's Hospital where he performed surgery.

One summer, he obtained a job for me as an elevator operator at Saint Luke's, where, in uniform and white gloves, I experienced a taste of hospital culture as I interacted with doctors, interns, nurses, patients, as well as the contrary folding metal elevator door. Later, my father opened an additional office in our home in Bronxville, and he also operated at the Laurence Hospital, working almost continuously, performing operations early in the morning, driving back and forth to New York, and seeing patients at both locations, along with making house calls.

In the 1930s, antibiotics were not available, and infections were often poorly controlled: my father often drained infected sinuses through the nose, surgically removed tonsils, and frequently performed operations on the mastoid bone, located in the skull behind the ear where infections spreading from the ear could endanger the brain. In this type of surgery, it was sometimes necessary to open the mastoid bone and curette it free of infection. I am told that he was very talented as a surgeon, able to operate using either hand with equal skill. Despite his place of residence, my father was never a "society doctor," catering primarily to the wealthy. Both in Bronxville and in New York City, he always had a number of patients who paid him very little or nothing, or paid him later, "when some money came in." Although prosperous, he never became very wealthy (unlike many of his colleagues); he was more interested in working hard in the profession he loved and in maintaining the respect of his patients and colleagues. He was a rather distant figure to me, but surely a worthy role model.

John Ross was a man of few words, particularly in his communications with me and with my older sister, Elizabeth (Betsy) Ross. He had a remarkable sense of humor and great rapport with his patients (except with dedicated smokers during World War II, when cigarettes, which he considered very damaging to the ears, nose, throat, and lungs, were scarce: he would often confiscate cigarette packages and throw them away. Needless to say, my sister and I were never allowed to smoke).

On Sundays, he used to put on his old clothes and work in our yard. As he told it, one day a lady came by in a large Cadillac, stopped, and said she would pay him a dollar more an hour than he was earning there.

He replied, "Well, thanks, but I think I'll just stay on here…you see the lady here lets me sleep with her." The woman drove off in a huff.

I am sure that my decision early in high school to become a doctor primarily grew out of my medical experiences with my father (perhaps as well as my desire to find some ground on which I might communicate with him), and also by my mother's frequent statements to her friends that "Johnny wants to be a doctor" (although she usually had not the slightest idea of what was going on inside my head).

My mother differed from my father in many ways. She was of more elevated socio-economic upbringing and raised initially in Kentucky, where her father, George Byron Moulder, was a landscape architect. He was among the early mail order entrepreneurs, raising and selling water lilies to Queen Victoria and others in the late nineteenth century. Later, he was in charge of landscaping the railroad stations for several rail lines. He moved the family to Nashville in 1917, and my mother attended Ward Belmont College and then studied piano and classical music at a conservatory in Chicago; she also played piano accompaniments in theaters for silent movies. After she and my father married, they initially settled in New York City, and when my sister and I were born, the family moved to Bronxville, in Westchester County, New York. There, my mother held dinners for physicians and their wives, which was important for the patient referral network and may also have been one of their motivations for joining so many (perhaps too many) private clubs: the Siwanoy Country Club (where my father golfed once a week, and where my mother golfed more frequently with her friends), the Bronxville Field Club (swimming, tennis, bowling, squash, and dinners and dances) for children and adults, the Shenarock Shore Club on Long Island

Sound, the Bronxville Women's Club (where my mother gave piano concerts and met with her music sorority), and the University Club in New York City. Later, my mother gave piano lessons at our home (possibly to help pay for a new Mason Hamlin grand piano and all those club memberships). My sister and I took piano lessons from another teacher, a musically gifted friend of the family.

Distant Lineages

In addition to her numerous club activities, my mother had an uncommon interest in ancestors, particularly her own. She became a member of the Daughters of the American Revolution (the DAR), which formally traced her direct descent, through family Bibles, church ledgers, and Revolutionary War records (1775–1783) in Washington, DC, through her mother, Eva Knowles, back to Permelia Greene, the sister of General Nathaniel Greene of Revolutionary War renown. Permelia married one Captain Matthew Smith of the Continental Army, also known as "Praying Matthew Smith" because he had lost both legs below the knee in the war and moved about with difficulty. All this was sufficient evidence for the DAR to award her membership. The DAR also checked out the Moulders (her father's line), only to discover that two early brothers in his direct lineage had traded with the British during the Revolution and later had some legal difficulties.

My mother also managed to trace my father's roots, so that he could join the Sons of the American Revolution (SAR). However, it was discovered that several generations of Rosses, including his father's father (John Ross, born in 1807) and an earlier James Ross, apparently lacked Revolutionary War zeal and did not serve in the army. However, my father's birth mother, Margaret Tennessee Armstrong, through her mother's line (the Tullochs) traced her lineage back to Magnus Tulloch, who was born in Scotland and at a tender age served in the American Revolution as a piper.

My father was highly skeptical of all this and, in the end, wanted nothing to do with the SAR. My mother did have success with my sister who became a DAR and later tried to sell me on the idea of joining the SAR, but I told her that I wanted no connection with a group that would not allow the great black singer Marion Anderson to sing at their hallowed Constitution Hall in Washington, DC.

Enough of lineages.

Every summer, from when I was three years old until I was ten, my mother would desert my father for about six weeks and journey by train with my sister and me to Nashville, Tennessee, to visit her family. During those summers, I became close to my grandfather, George Byron Moulder, and in that period, the 1930s, there was an efflorescence of public parks in Nashville. Mr. Moulder, as a landscape architect, became superintendent of parks for the city. The parks were built by the WPA (Works Project Administration) workers supported by President Franklin Delano Roosevelt, and with additional philanthropic support from the Warner family of Nashville; Percy Warner Park was a popular picnic area.

My grandfather was also involved in and published a small book about the reconstruction in Nashville of a perfect replica, and therefore built with only curved lines, of the original Parthenon in Greece (completed in 458 BC). The replica had been originally constructed for the 1897 Centennial Exposition in Nashville, and it was rebuilt in concrete between 1920 and 1930 (fig. 1); it contained a replica of the original statue of Athena from the Greek Parthenon (fig. 2). With my grandfather, I frequented this building, which stands today in

Nashville's Centennial Park. During those years, as I traveled with him to various construction sites, I decided that I wanted to become an architect. I have maintained a strong interest in architecture, but this career inclination was swamped with later interests and family pressures toward medicine.

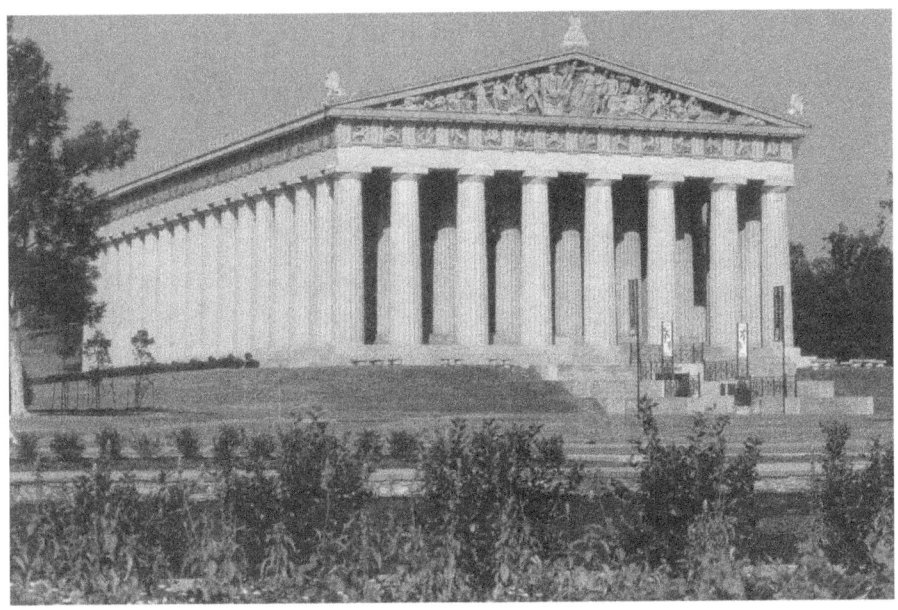

Figure 1. The Parthenon. Nashville, Tennessee
(Replica of the original in Athens, Greece)

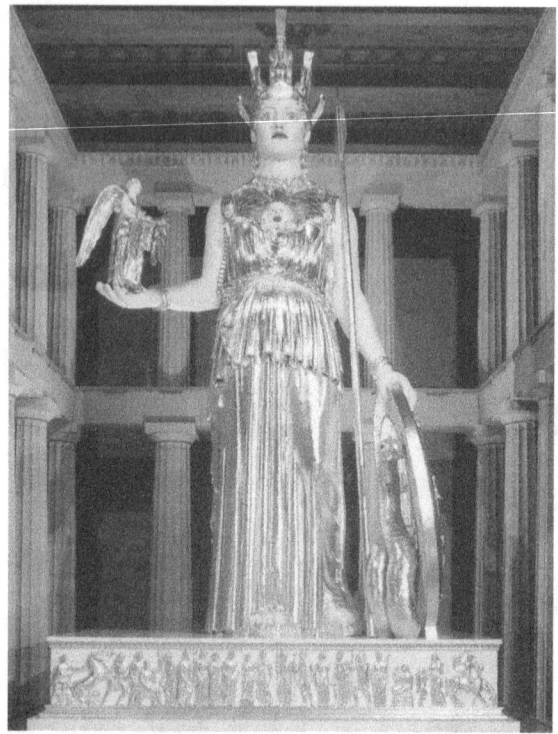

Figure 2. Athena. Nashville, Tennessee
(Replica of the original in Athens, Greece)

More on Bronxville

A small, tightly knit, exclusive (indeed exclusionary) community, Bronxville had a fine public school that was well supported by state and high local taxes. The Bronxville School was attended, with few exceptions, by Bronxville residents (a few fortunate souls in neighboring communities were allowed to enter, but were considered by some to be from the other side of the tracks). The school was (and still is) a large brick structure of Tudor style architecture. It housed classes from kindergarten through the twelfth grade, which most of my classmates and I attended for all thirteen years. A modest number of students dropped out in the ninth grade to attend college preparatory (prep) schools such as Andover, Taft, and Groton, but my father considered the Bronxville School perfectly adequate. I did well scholastically there, played football, and was elected senior class president.

The teachers in the Bronxville School were excellent and generally well paid. Social life was active, and so-called romances sometimes began in the second grade (I had one of those when Annie M. declared herself my girlfriend). To a large degree, Bronxville boys and girls grew up together throughout grade school and high school. In fact, liaisons in high school not uncommonly ended in marriages after college. In addition, the Bronxville High School had an excellent record of college placements, helped no doubt by the extensive social and business connections of most of the parents. I ended up in the Ivy League at Dartmouth College in Hanover, New Hampshire, where I majored in the premedical curriculum (chemistry-zoology).

High Society

It was considered desirable for Bronxville girls to have a debut (my older sister attended a joint debut at which she and a number of her contemporaries were "presented" to society). I also attended some debuts where only one girl was presented. Such debuts were always followed by a ball, complete with champagne and a "society orchestra" (usually Lester Lanin). Such events in Bronxville were relatively conservative, unlike the lavish affairs held for famous debutantes in New York City.

Our entrée into high society was facilitated by Miss Covington's dance lessons. In her classes, attended by many of us between the ages of ten and fifteen, Miss Covington was an imposing figure in the full bloom of late middle age; she was always attired in a full-length evening dress, her figure enhanced and supported (I was sure) by a Victorian corset. Wearing midheel dancing slippers with straps, lifting her gown slightly, she would glide with remarkable grace across the floor demonstrating dance steps. A strict disciplinarian, she carried a clicker, using it on the slightest provocation to maintain order. Each weekly class held during the winter season was composed of an equal number of boys and girls, who convened for several months at the Hotel Gramatan (named after an historic American Indian chief). We would be seated, boys on one side of the room, and white-gloved girls on the other. After her lecture (which always included comments on social etiquette) and her demonstration, it came time for us to dance: the boys would invite the girls seated opposite them across the room to partner. Then, Miss Covington's assistant, Miss Darupel, would provide the appropriate music on a large grand piano. Dancing was exclusively in formal ballroom style; boys placed their open right hand on their partner's back while holding her right hand up with his left hand, and she, in turn, resting her weightless left hand on his right shoulder—"Girls, you must never drag down on his shoulder"—as the dance commenced on the proper beat. In this way we learned the foxtrot and the waltz, progressing to the rhumba, the tango and, as a special treat, an occasional, sedate jitterbug. Later, in high school, at the same hotel in which our dance classes were held, an annual dress ball was hosted by the "Bronxville Bachelors," an organization of obscure origins of which I was a member.

Of course, it was considered highly desirable that young Bronxville men, during or soon after college, marry Bronxville girls (preferably from appropriately moneyed families). I had escaped this fate by leaving for college and immediately after college attending medical school, never returning to live in Bronxville. Indeed, when, after my internship and a period of research at the National Institutes of Health, I decided to marry an outsider, there was considerable disappointment in my family. Twelve years after our marriage, when I left my first wife after discovering that she was a secret alcoholic, my mother renewed her long held hope that I would finally marry a Bronxville girl and settle down in a medical practice near home. Once again her hopes proved fruitless.

By that time, I had become an academic in California, where I met another academic, Lola Romanucci, an anthropologist, who later became Lola Romanucci-Ross, the love of my life. Having both experienced unhappy first marriages, we commenced our first "real" marriage with each other. When I first took Lola to Bronxville to meet my family, my mother introduced her to some of the Bronxville ladies. Upon learning that she was of Italian descent (second generation, born in Hershey, Pennsylvania), they cheerfully chirped that they actually *knew* some Italians: there was Mr. Panetieri the grocer, Mr. Duletto the tailor and Ettore Barone the gardener. I said, "*This* Italian is different. She is a professor of anthropology at my university, the University of California San Diego (UCSD)." The ladies became properly muted, but Lola accepted my mother and her lady friends gracefully, and later she expressed mild amusement to me, noting that despite their frequent trips to tour Italy, these Bronxvillians did not seem to connect their admiration of Italian science, art, architecture, music, and fine cuisine to the Italian people who created it.

Varieties of Religious Experience

There were several churches in Bronxville, including Roman Catholic, Episcopal, and Presbyterian, as well as Christian Science. However, Bronxville's religious affiliations were impacted by its seventeenth-century founder, the Dutchman, Johannes Bronk. Bronk arrived before the British came, when New York was called New Amsterdam. He also founded the part of New York City just north of Manhattan Island, known as "the Bronx" (an area housing a mixture of immigrant peoples, and from which Bronxville residents always took pains to disassociate their town.) In any case, one holdover from the Dutch "occupation" was the Dutch Reformed Church, a large Romanesque stone structure complete with cloister, a large central nave, classrooms, a bell tower and a magnificent pipe organ (played from time to time by the famed organist E. Power Biggs). The church still stands, across from the Bronxville town library. My mother and father had agreed when they married that my father would discontinue his membership in the Baptist Church but remain an East Tennessee Republican, and that my mother would release her tie to the Presbyterian Church and change her allegiance from the Democratic to the Republican Party.

On Sundays, my family would attend the service at the Dutch Reformed Church, listen to the sermon, sing hymns, and hear the organ and choir music; after the service, my sister and I would attend Sunday school. I must confess that my boredom during the church service was extreme; I would study the stained glass windows and invent stories to go with the scenes, read the Hymn Book hoping to find anything at all of interest, and scrutinize the faces of the other worshippers, sometimes making eye contact with a kindred bored spirit. That all changed when a new minister took over. The Reverend J.P. was a handsome younger man whose sermons were dynamic and full of ideas and philosophy. He became an instant success with me and with many others in the congregation, particularly the women, and he mixed socially with Bronxville's upper crust. It later came to light that the Reverend had been having an affair with one of the wives in his congregation, and his tenure thereafter was short-lived, much to my disappointment.

A lasting impact of my church involvement included my experience with an elderly dowager scion of Bronxville, Miss Amy Dusenberry (with emphasis on the *Miss*), who lived alone in a colonial mansion dating back to the Revolutionary War. Miss Amy was active in our church, and she invited eight young men from among Bronxville High School juniors and seniors to become members of her Board of Directors, "The Board of Directors of the Greatest Business in the World, the Business of Living Life as Christ Taught It." I was among those chosen. Miss Amy held regular meetings with us at the Dutch Reformed Church, where we would discuss a broad range of topics, hear her views, and offer our own on how we could and should have a positive impact within and outside the community. We would undertake an occasional project, such as helping to feed the poor in surrounding areas, but her major effect on me was the example of her strong character and her vision of what constitutes good moral behavior.

An Unlikely Encounter, with a Happy Ending

By my description of Bronxville's somewhat narrow-minded culture, I do not mean to disparage the good people of Bronxville or their way of life. The community in which I lived for so many formative and happy years was certainly well ordered; here life was almost preordained, nothing was lacking, and a comfortable road lay ahead. But as I left for college and then medical school, I felt certain that I would never want to enter private practice, particularly in an area where I could probably do well professionally and financially, but in which I was not really needed. There must be something more meaningful to undertake,

I thought, something that would enhance knowledge about the complex functions of the organs of the human body in health and disease and be brought to bear cognitively on developing better forms of diagnosis and treatment.

At about the same stage of her life, Lola Romanucci had decided that she wanted to leave the place where she grew up, Hershey, Pennsylvania, and turn herself outward toward the world, in her case to become an anthropologist in order to study other peoples and cultures. So, too, did I want to leave home, but my urge was to focus my gaze inward to understand the human body, how normal physiologic function can become deranged, and how to diagnose and treat bodily dysfunctions. Given the different directions of our two upbringings and careers, it was unlikely that our paths would ever cross. But, thanks to the umbrella of a large university, the University of California San Diego at which we both became professors, they finally did, and in 1972 Lola became Lola Romanucci-Ross. Later, we discovered that two disparate professional pathways, the study of man in his culture, and the human body in its environment, had many points of complementarity, and we have been talking, writing, and in love ever since.

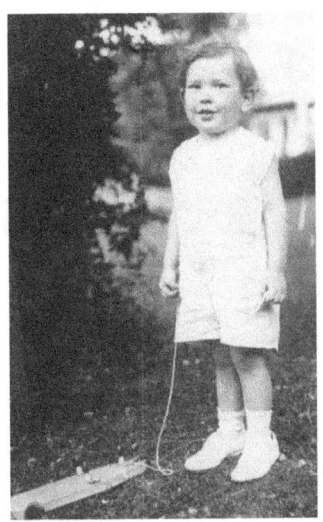

Figure 3.

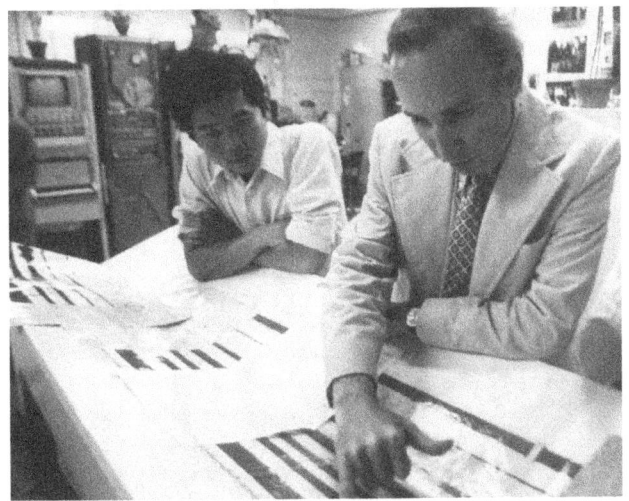

Figure 4.

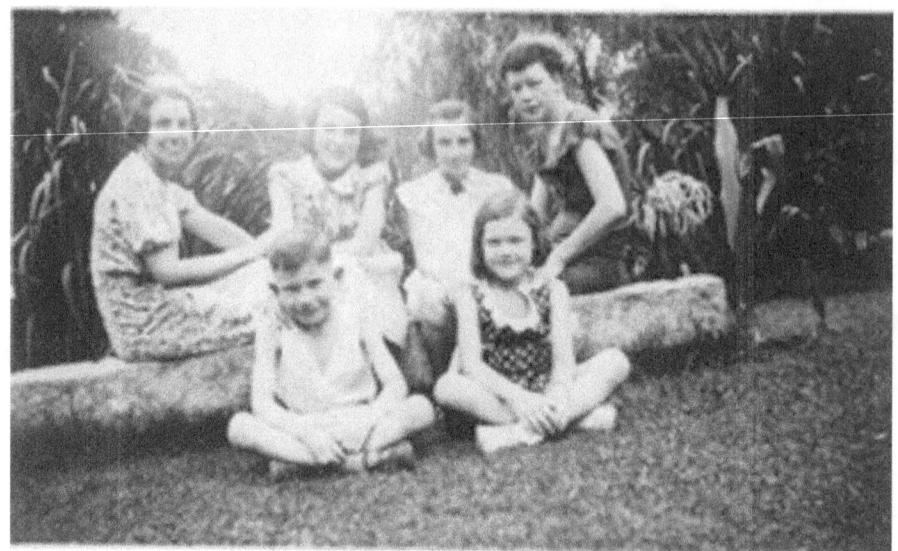

Figure 5.

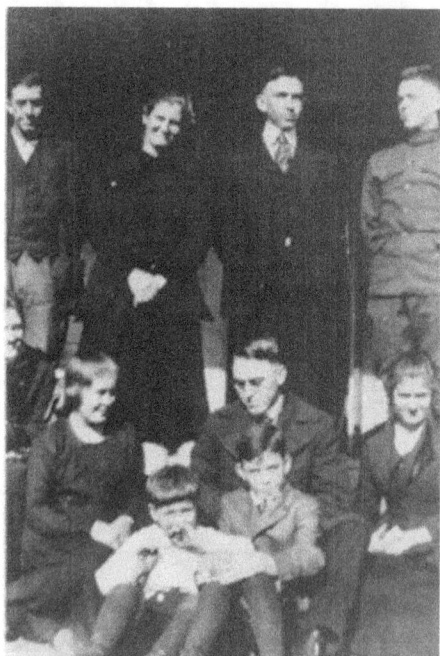

Figure 6.

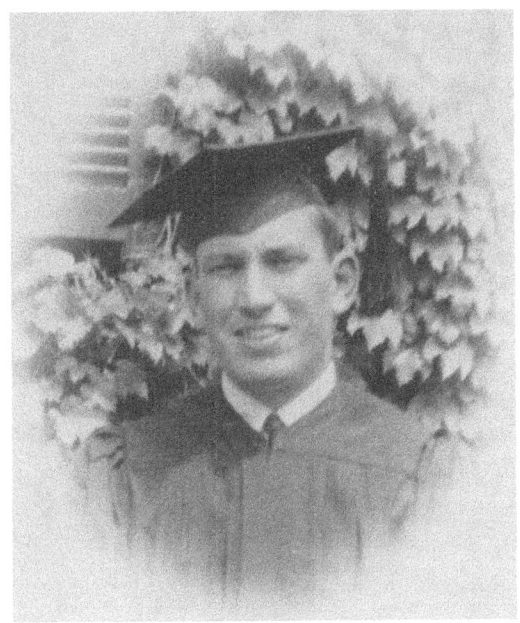

Figure 7.

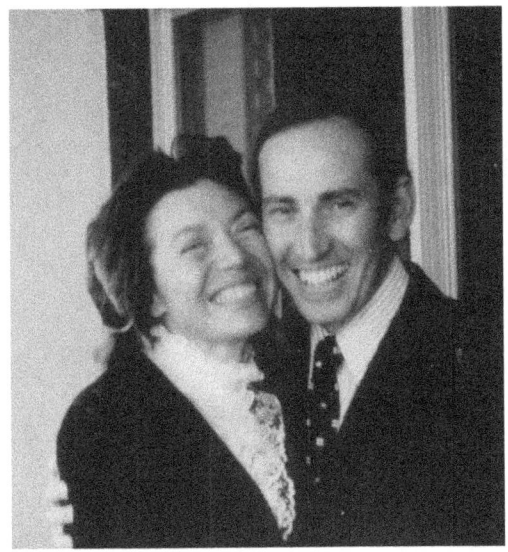

Figure 8.

CHAPTER 2
INTO THE SUBCULTURE OF MEDICINE

My medical-scientific career began in 1951 at the Cornell University College of Medicine (now Weill Cornell Medical College) in New York City (class of 1955) where, in my first-year class in biochemistry, we learned about nucleic acids, including deoxyribose nucleic acid (DNA). However, there was no discussion of the function or significance of DNA structure, even though three years earlier Watson and Crick[1] had published their groundbreaking model of DNA structure and its implications for genetic transmission, a testimonial to the lag from discovery to dispersion of scientific knowledge in those times.

My career trajectory was established during my subsequent internship in surgery at the Johns Hopkins Hospital, where I studied under Dr. Alfred Blalock, professor of surgery and famed creator of the "blue baby" operation along with pediatrician Dr. Helen Taussig. This operation was performed on babies with cyanotic heart disease and involved

---

1 JD Watson and F. Crick, "Molecular Structure of Nucleic Acids: A Structure for Deoxyribose Nucleic Acid." *Nature* 171 (1953): 737–738.

attaching the subclavian artery of the arm to the pulmonary artery, a procedure that improved blood flow to the lungs and enhanced delivery of oxygenated blood to the rest of the body, thereby "turning blue babies pink."[2]

Drs. Blalock and Taussig joined a succession of distinguished physicians who began a tradition of scientific medicine at Johns Hopkins, and whose careers and accomplishments led me to read avidly about that history during the few moments I could spare from my duties as an intern. The founding of the Johns Hopkins Medical School in 1893 was a major turning point in medical education in the United States, marking the beginning of an era of scientific medicine in this country, although many of the new practices were already in use in German medical schools, and some had been in place at the Italian medical school at Salerno beginning in the ninth century.

An outstanding faculty of clinical scholars and investigators was recruited to Hopkins soon after the founding of the medical school, among them Sir William Osler, who became professor of medicine and physician-in-chief of the Johns Hopkins Hospital. Osler was the first to describe several diseases, and he produced a classic textbook of medicine. Also recruited was William Halsted as professor of surgery, who devised several new operations and perfected aseptic surgical techniques, including the use of sterilized rubber gloves and fine black silk sutures.

A Side Trip into History

Stimulated by the historical ambiance at Hopkins and the focus on cardiac surgery by Dr. Blalock, I bought several used books concerned

---

[2] A Blalock and B Taussig, "The Surgical Treatment of Malformations of the Heart in Which There is Pulmonary Stenosis or Pulmonary Atresia. *JAMA* 128, no. 3 (1945):189–202.

with the history of medicine, and whenever some free time was available, I delved into early descriptions of the heart and circulation. I learned that the heart received scant mention in early Egyptian writings, nor was it a theme in the therapies described by the Greek physician Hippocrates (460–370 BC), who has been called the father of medicine.[3] Aristotle described the anatomy of the heart in several animal species, and he noted the movement of the human fetal heart.[4] Later, much of Greek medicine was imported to Rome, where the famous Greek physician Galen (131–201 AD) practiced medicine for many years. Galen also developed a number of theories and doctrines, some of which dominated medical and scientific thought until the beginning of the Renaissance in the sixteenth century. Among these doctrines was Galen's view that the movement of blood in the human body could be considered to ebb and flow backward and forward within both the arteries and the veins, which he considered to have no direct connection with each other.[5] Rather, he believed there were invisible pores in the partition (septum) between the two ventricles of the heart through which blood could pass from the right to the left side of the circulation.

The detailed anatomic dissections and drawings of the human body by Andreas Vesalius (1514–64) began to dismantle many of Galen's doctrines. Vesalius, who was Flemish, of German extraction, was the public prosecutor in Padua (Padova) Italy, a famous center of learning in that period. There, for a number of years, he extensively dissected human corpses with his students and carefully described the structure of various organs in their natural position. The anatomic studies of the heart

---

[3] Greek Medicine-The Hippocratic Oath. National Institutes of Health, US National Library of Medicine.
[4] E. Crivellato and D. Ribatti, "A portrait of Aristotle as an anatomist: historical article," *Clinical Anatomy* 20, no. 5 (2007):447–85.
[5] F. H. Garrison. *An introduction to the history of medicine: with medical chronology, suggestions for study and bibliographic data*, 4th ed. (Philadelphia: W.B. Saunders Company, 1929).

by Vesalius included descriptions of the heart valves and the coronary arteries, providing the basis for modern knowledge of cardiac anatomy (see his book *De Fabrica Humani Corporis*).[6]

In the seventeenth century, Englishman William Harvey (1578–1657), completed the destruction of Galenic ideas about circulation by learning that blood moves continuously around in circulation. Harvey, also working at the University of Padova some years after Vesalius, found that Italian anatomists had described one-way valves in the veins, and he carried out a series of experiments in animals in which he was able to calculate the output of blood from the heart by use of selective ligatures and timed collections of blood; he also estimated the total volume of blood contained in circulation. These and other experiments allowed Harvey to demonstrate conclusively that the only possible way that the output of blood by the heart could be maintained was if blood recirculated continuously.[7] But exactly how such recirculation could be accomplished awaited discovery of the microscope.

Vesalius had demonstrated the close proximity of the ends of small arteries and the origins of small veins, but it was the Italian microscopist Marcello Malpighi (1628–1694) who first described tiny blood vessels surrounding the air sacs in the lungs. These short, very thin-walled blood vessels (capillaries) have a diameter not much larger than that of a red blood cell (seven to eight millionths of a meter, or 8 microns). Later, capillaries were found in organs throughout the body, where they serve to supply nutrients and allow gas exchange (oxygen delivery and carbon dioxide removal) in the tissues.

---

6 A. Vesalius, *De humani corporis fabrica libri septem. Basileae: Ex officinal Joannis Oporini*. (1543).
7 W. Harvey, *Exercitatio anatomica de motu cordis et sanguinis in animalibus*. (Frankfurt: William Fitzer. 1628).

The capillaries of the body are so numerous that their total cross-sectional area in various organs and tissues can readily accommodate the entire cardiac output as it is pumped by the right ventricle through the lungs, where venous blood is reoxygenated and cleared of carbon dioxide before being returned to the left atrium and then to the left ventricle, which pumps it into the aorta. From the aorta the freshly oxygenated blood is distributed to the numerous smaller arteries of the body, which direct flow to the capillary beds of the brain, the heart, the limbs, and various organs in the abdomen.

This historical review was of great interest to me, but the time had come for me to begin my official clinical training, so I undertook the first rung of this ladder, an internship. I decided to start with a surgical one.

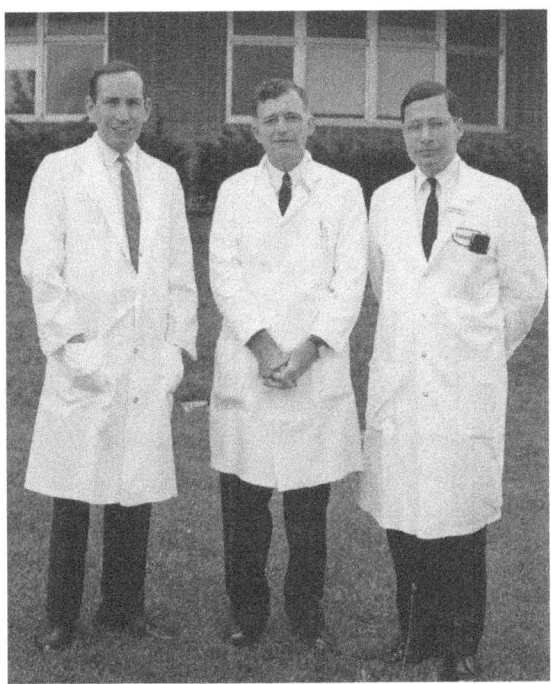

Figure 9.

CHAPTER 3
INTERNSHIP AND A MOVE TO THE NATIONAL INSTITUTES OF HEALTH

What, exactly, were the duties of a surgical intern at the Johns Hopkins Hospital in 1956 when I had just graduated from the School of Medicine at Cornell? I soon learned that interns were paid twenty-five dollars per month (a pittance even then) and were not permitted to leave the hospital at any time, unless all patients on their services were stable and had adequate medical coverage. The surgical interns were to interview, examine, and write-up all patients admitted to the hospital for surgical procedures, both those admitted to rooms on the "private service" and those placed on the wards as "charity patients." We rotated monthly to the surgical subspecialties, including general surgery (mainly of the abdomen), urology, ophthalmology, ear, nose, and throat, plastic surgery, cardiac, and thoracic surgery.

We also served frequent shifts in the accident room (known as "The Ax"). There, we encountered and treated (under supervision) all sorts of acute medical emergencies. The Johns Hopkins Hospital, in those days, was located in the midst of a rough, economically depressed section of Baltimore, and knife wounds to the chest, heart, abdomen, and limbs were common. In some cases, a knife wound to the chest would penetrate the heart, often causing copious bleeding from the heart into the pericardial sac around the heart, which could produce cardiac tamponade and required immediate drainage by inserting a small tube through the chest wall into the pericardial sac. We also encountered many cases of severe alcohol intoxication known as the "DTs" (*delirium tremens*).

In such a bustling, hectic environment, a meaningful encounter with Dr. Blalock was a stellar event for me. In the operating room, Dr. Blalock complained constantly about the insufficient assistance he received, particularly from interns and nurses (his usual whining comment: "won't *somebody* help me?"). On one occasion, I was "scrubbed in" with him and several more senior assistants. As a lowly surgical intern, I was thrilled when Dr. Blalock asked me to help him tighten the long, running stitch at the back of a surgical connection created by attaching the end of the subclavian artery of the arm to a branch of the pulmonary artery leading to the lungs, in order to improve blood flow to the lungs in children with cyanosis. Usually such blue babies are a consequence of several birth defects causing inadequate flow of blood to the lungs; these defects included narrowing of the valve in the pulmonary artery leading to the lungs and an abnormal shunt of venous blood (blue, deoxygenated blood) into the left side of the heart through a congenital defect in the septum separating the two ventricles. In the surgical procedure devised by Drs. Blalock and Taussig, the artificial shunt of oxygenated blood to the lungs, produced by attaching the subclavian artery of the arm to the pulmonary artery leading to the lungs, blood flow to the lungs increased, relieving the "blue" condition and making possible relatively normal growth and activity of an otherwise severely limited baby.[8]

With the later advent of open heart surgery, it became possible to directly repair all the cardiac abnormalities in most of these babies, many of whom had "Tetralogy of Fallot." so named after the French physician who first described four congenital heart defects: narrowing of the valve in the pulmonary artery leading to the lungs (pulmonic stenosis), a ventricular septal defect (a hole in the wall dividing the left and right ventricles), an aorta that overrides the defect in the ventricular septum, and enlargement of the right ventricle.[9]

A Change in Venue: On to the National Heart Institute

At the end of the internship year, I was one of two surgical interns among the twelve in our group who where invited to go to the then National Heart Institute of the National Institutes of Health (NIH) in Bethesda, Maryland, a one hour's drive south of Baltimore. There we were to receive two years of training in cardiac surgery and to perform cardiovascular research. Arriving fresh from an internship in the large academic teaching hospital at Johns Hopkins, I found myself in the milieu of a very large research institute. The initial culture shock was soon transformed into excitement and eagerness to learn and perform. Many of the Institutes had clinical services for patients involved in research protocols at the NIH Clinical Center, and as a clinical associate in the Clinic of Surgery, I was assigned duties on the inpatient ward involving the diagnosis and post-operative care of patients with congenital and

---

[8] A. Blalock and B. Taussig, "The surgical treatment of malformations of the heart in which there is pulmonary stenosis or pulmonary atresia." *JAMA* 128, no. 3 (1945): 189–202.

[9] Blalock and Taussig, "Surgical treatment of malformations," 189–202.

acquired heart disease who were candidates for surgical treatment. Also, I was expected to undertake both clinical and laboratory research, the latter to include studies in experimental animals in an adjacent building.

Dr. Andrew "Glenn" Morrow, chief of the clinic of surgery of the National Heart Institute, had trained in cardiac surgery at the Johns Hopkins Hospital under Dr. Blalock. He was interested in developing new diagnostic and surgical methods for the management of patients with acquired or congenital heart disease. In 1956, heart-lung machines were being developed to support circulation and thereby allow open-heart surgery to be performed. Dr. Morrow was interested in evaluating the new Melrose pump-oxygenator, designed and fabricated in England by Dr. Dennis Melrose who came to our clinic to demonstrate its use. The device had a large rolling plastic drum containing multiple internal fins to film and oxygenate the blood, along with compression pumps with valves to propel the blood. This system proved to be problematic, largely because of air bubble formation.

I first worked in research with Dr. Robert Bowman, chief of the laboratory of technical development at the NIH, in an effort to develop an oxygenator that used a series of thin plastic membranes, so that blood could be oxygenated without direct contact between gas and blood. However, I was unable to construct such a system that would allow a sufficiently high blood flow to be useful in adult patients. Subsequently, working primarily with a fellow trainee, Dr. John Waldhausen, we used a device fabricated to film and oxygenate blood in an enclosed, oxygen-rich atmosphere. This device was used successfully and safely in a number of patients for open-heart operations. Still later, the so-called bubble oxygenator, which efficiently produced and then removed gaseous oxygen bubbles, proved to be more efficient and came into wide use.

INTERNSHIP AND A MOVE TO THE NATIONAL INSTITUTES OF HEALTH

However, rather than device development, it was the physiologically oriented laboratory research that could be translated to patient care that held the greatest interest for me. This occupied most of my subsequent research time, so I stayed on at the NIH as a senior investigator in the Clinic of Surgery for an additional two years beyond my original assignment in order to learn more about the relatively new technique of cardiac catheterization.

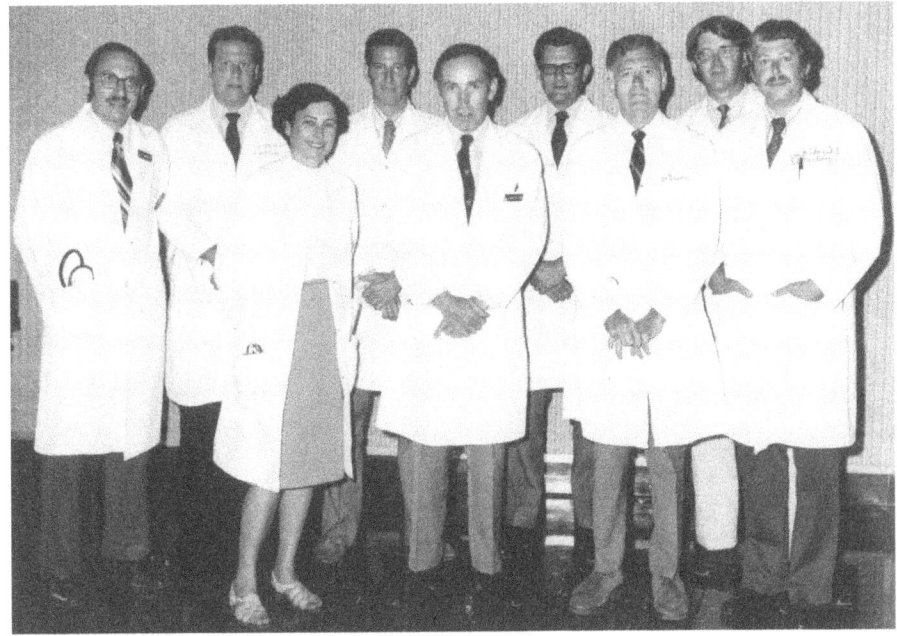

Figure 10.

CHAPTER 4
CARDIAC CATHETERIZATION

Catheterization of the Right Heart

For centuries, Egyptians and Greeks performed explorations of all the chambers of the human heart only after death, and Galen offered subsequent descriptions of the four heart chambers.[10] Later, the detailed anatomic dissections and drawings of Vesalius (1560) provided the basis for modern knowledge of heart structure, including the heart valves, the anatomy of the small blood vessels that supply blood to the heart muscle, and the coronary arteries.[11] However, it was not until the twentieth century that visualization of hearts in living human subjects, and the determination of pressures and blood flows inside the cardiac chambers, became feasible.

In 1929, a German intern, Werner Forssmann, first performed catheterization of the right heart on himself, passing a urinary

---

10 F. H. Garrison, *An introduction to the history of medicine: with medical chronology, suggestions for study and bibliographic data*, 4th ed. (Philadelphia: W.B. Saunders Company, 1929).

11 A. Vesalius, *De humani corporis fabrica libri septem. Basileae: Ex officinal Joannis Oporini.* (1543).

catheter, which was opaque to X rays, through a vein all the way into the receiving chamber of the right heart (the right atrium) where he drew a blood sample and took an X ray of the catheter within the heart.

Later, two physicians in New York, Andre Cournand and Dickinson Richards, went further, passing a long thin catheter visible on fluoroscopy from the right atrium into the right ventricle (the pumping chamber of the right heart) and then further into the pulmonary artery, measuring pressures at each location and drawing blood samples used for calculating the blood flow rate (the cardiac output). Subsequently, many such measurements were found to be abnormal in patients with heart disease. For these accomplishments Forssmann, Cournand, and Richards received the 1956 Nobel Prize in Medicine and Physiology. The catheterization procedure was painless for the patient, since the lining of the blood vessels and the heart chambers does not contain nerve receptors for pain or touch.

As clinical associates at the National Heart Institute, we were responsible for performing diagnostic cardiac catheterizations in patients admitted to the NIH Clinical Center for evaluation of their heart disorders. At that time (1956), right heart catheterization had been developed relatively recently and involved the use of a small plastic tube called a catheter (two to three feet in length and opaque to X rays), which could be observed under a fluoroscope. The catheter was inserted into a vein through a small incision in the arm in front of the elbow, and the tip of the catheter was then maneuvered within the vein into the larger veins of the chest, where it could be observed on a fluoroscopic screen. When I began to perform right heart cardiac catheterizations in 1956, fluoroscopes were not very efficient, and it was necessary to wear goggles with red lenses for a number of minutes to allow adaptation to the dark before beginning the procedure. Accordingly, we worked in semidarkness with a high-intensity X ray to see the heart and the catheter on the fluoroscopic screen. These problems were eliminated several years later by the development of efficient X ray image intensifiers, which greatly improved the images of the heart while emitting much less radiation to the patient (and the physician).

A number of disorders of the heart can be present at birth (congenital malformations), and most of these heart defects can be detected by right heart catheterization in children of all ages, as well as in individuals who survive to adulthood. I became adept at many of the procedures that aided such detection. For example, if there is a hole (a defect) in the septum dividing the two sides of the heart between either the atria (an atrial septal defect) or the ventricles (a ventricular septal defect), the higher pressure normally present in the left heart causes a shunt of oxygenated blood from left to right. In this setting, drawing a series of blood samples from the vena cava, the right atrium, the right ventricle, and the pulmonary artery will reveal the location of the shunt (high oxygen content in the right atrium due to an atrial septal defect, or in the right ventricle due to a ventricular septal defect), or, if there is an abnormal connection between the aorta and the pulmonary artery (patent ductus arteriosus), the blood oxygen content will be high only in the pulmonary artery. Drawing blood samples from multiple locations allows calculation of the magnitude of the abnormal left to right shunt of blood. Measuring pressure in the right ventricle and pulmonary artery can reveal high pressures in both locations due to a large left to right shunt, or in the right ventricle alone due to congenital narrowing of the pulmonic valve with low pressure in the pulmonary artery. Angiography can reveal narrowing either within the right ventricle or at the pulmonic valve.

Another procedure used in right heart catheterization allowed an estimation of the pressure in the receiving chamber of the left heart (the left atrium). Forcing the tip of a catheter into a small pulmonary artery results in transmission of a somewhat distorted left atrial pressure waves across the lung capillaries. Elevation of this so-called wedge pressure (which is now measured by inflating a small balloon attached to a catheter in a branch of the pulmonary artery) may reflect heart failure or disease of the valves in the left heart. I, and other physicians training in the Clinic of Surgery, performed all of these diagnostic procedures in patients with complex heart malformations, or in those with disease of one or more cardiac valves, prior to considering surgical corrections.

Coronary Angiography

In the late 1960s and the early 1970s, angiography of the coronary arteries was developed, and it was found that a very common cause of left ventricular dysfunction or heart failure was coronary atherosclerosis causing narrowing or occlusion of one or more coronary arteries. Initially, the coronary arteries were visualized by injecting X ray contrast medium into the root of the aorta. Later, injection of X ray contrast liquid directly into each coronary artery using a catheter inserted through the arm or leg while recording X ray motion pictures allowed precise delineation of atherosclerotic plaques in the coronary arteries, an approach refined by Dr. F. Mason Sones of the Cleveland Clinic. Such plaques, if severe enough to produce chest pain during exercise (angina pectoris), may then be treated by coronary artery bypass surgery or by percutaneous coronary balloon angioplasty (PTCA), the latter often followed by placement of an expandable metal device within the artery (a stent), to keep the vessel open.

Catheterization of the Left Heart

Disorders affecting the left-sided chambers of the heart in adult patients include diseases of the mitral and aortic valves accompanied by narrowing or leakage of one or both of the valves due to scarring caused by rheumatic fever or to congenital abnormalities, including narrowing of the aortic valve, which tend to become increasingly severe later in life. Enlargement and failure of the muscle cells of the main pumping chamber of the heart, the left ventricle, may occur due to longstanding overload on the heart caused by aortic or mitral valve disease, or to high blood pressure (hypertension), which can result in similar failure of the left ventricular heart muscle. Primary myocardial disease (cardiomyopathy) usually of unknown cause can also cause such failure.

In the 1950s and early 1960s, the main focus of cardiac catheterization in adults was to characterize disorders of the valves, and to identify primary and secondary disease of the heart muscle.

Transbronchial Left Heart Catheterization

Dr. Andrew "Glenn" Morrow, of the NIH, frequently used an approach for measuring pressures and blood flow in the left side of the heart, where disease of the mitral and aortic valves required evaluation of their severity and the potential for surgical treatment. Such disease caused abnormalities of the pressures within the left atrium and the left ventricle (the receiving and pumping chambers, respectively, of the left heart); it also sometimes caused reduced blood flow rates, which were also measured.

Transbronchial left heart catheterization[12] involved bronchoscopy insertion (after local tracheal anesthesia), of a rigid metal tube called a bronchoscope through the mouth and into the windpipe (trachea) in the conscious patient, who lay on his or her back. The far end of the bronchoscope was then positioned at the point where the trachea divides into two branches leading to the right and left lungs. The left atrium lies immediately adjacent to the start of the left main stem bronchus, and transbronchial catheterization involved passing a long needle down through the bronchoscope and puncturing through the wall of the bronchus in order to enter the adjacent left atrium. Pressure could then be recorded in that chamber, and a very small plastic tube could be advanced through the needle into the left atrium and then further into the left ventricle, where pressure was also measured and a dye was injected to measure blood flow (the cardiac output). This procedure, while relatively safe, was quite uncomfortable for the patient and necessarily brief. My role during this procedure was to stand next to Dr. Morrow holding a small length of plastic tubing, and to feed it to him as he tried to maneuver it from the left atrium into the left ventricle.

As I stood next to Dr. Morrow, I often thought to myself, *there must be a better way.*

My interest in developing a better method than the transbronchial approach for entering the left heart chambers, as well as other even riskier methods then in occasional use (such as passing a long needle

---

[12] A. Morrow, E. Braunwald, and J. Ross Jr., "Left heart catheterization: An Appraisal of Techniques and their Applications in Cardiovascular Diagnosis," *Arch Intern Med* 105 (1960): 645–655.

through the back, or the neck, to reach the left heart), led me to devise a new method that has since found a number of applications.

The Invention of Transseptal Left Heart Catheterization

One day, a visitor to the cardiac catheterization laboratory at the National Heart Institute of the NIH was watching me perform a right heart catheterization in a patient with an atrial septal defect. When I inserted the catheter through a vein in the leg, I passed it across the atrial septum through the defect to obtain pressures and blood samples from the left atrium and left ventricle. The visitor and I mused whether it might be possible to reach the left side of the heart when the atrial septum is intact.

That episode began my first personal research project. I asked the machine shop at the NIH to fabricate a long needle, which was curved at the distal end with a reverse bevel of the needle tip, and with a handle at the proximal end consisting of an attached metal arrow pointing in the direction of curve of the needle (fig. 11).

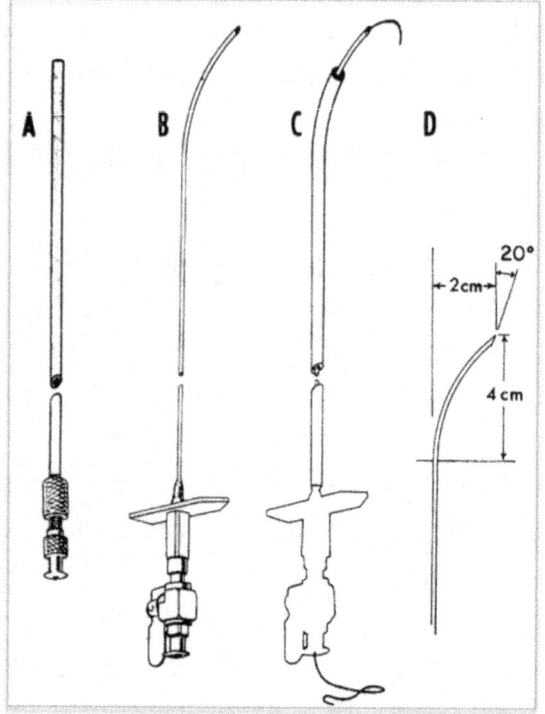

Figure 11. The original transseptal needle through which a small catheter could be passed to enter the left ventricle. Arch Intern Med. 1960;105:648.

I began experimenting with my instrument in studies in anesthetized animals under the fluoroscope. In this way, I engaged in a learning process for proper manipulation of the needle; this included allowing the needle to rotate when it was passed inside a cardiac catheter, after the tip of the catheter had been positioned in the right atrium. With the needle tip just inside the tip of the catheter, I used the metal handle to rotate the catheter tip to rest against the atrial septum. Since the needle was seven to eight millimeters longer than the catheter, when it was pushed forward, the septum was punctured. A blood sample was then drawn through the needle from the left atrium, and the sample was bright red (fully oxygenated) compared to the dark venous blood sample previously drawn from the right atrium. The pressure waves in the left atrium were then recorded, which differed from those in the right atrium, and I found that it was possible to pass a small plastic catheter through the needle (fig. 11, C) and to advance it across the mitral valve into the left ventricle, where the pressure was also recorded. This procedure was performed safely in a number of animals, and the small puncture site in the septum was found to fully heal in two to three weeks. In 1958, this early work on transseptal puncture in animals was published.[13]

I was eager to learn, of course, whether this approach could be translated into a procedure for use in humans. Therefore, soon after I established that the procedure was feasible and safe in animals, I approached the pathologist who performed autopsies at the NIH Clinical Center and asked if, after the chest was opened and he had completed his examination, but before the heart was removed, I might try my catheterization procedure. He agreed, and in the first of several such procedures in cadavers using a longer needle, I cut a large opening in the outside wall of the right atrium so that I could observe the atrial septum while standing at the right side of the chest. I then opened the saphenous vein in the upper right leg and passed a catheter upward toward the chest until the tip arrived in the right atrium. The curved needle was then inserted into the catheter, allowing it to rotate freely as it traveled upward until the needle tip lay just inside the catheter tip. Using the arrow-handle on the needle at the site of entry into the leg, the catheter and contained needle were rotated so that the tip lay firmly against the atrial septum. Since the needle was ten millimeters longer than the catheter, when the needle

---

[13] J. Ross Jr., "Catheterization of the left heart through the interatrial septum: a new technique and its experimental evaluation," *Surg Forum* 9 (1958): 297–300.

was pushed forward while holding the catheter in place, the septum was readily punctured.

Initial Studies in Patients Using the Transseptal Approach

The first patient studied was a young man with severe leakage of the mitral valve (mitral regurgitation) due to valvular scarring from rheumatic fever in childhood. His left atrium was greatly enlarged, and I could readily identify it under the fluoroscope; also, it was possible to feel the enlarged left atrium with the end of the catheter as it bulged into the right atrium.

With the head of the National Heart Institute's cardiology branch, Dr. Eugene Braunwald, and the head of the National Heart Institute's Clinic of Surgery, Dr. Morrow observing, I performed cardiac catheterization from the right leg and positioned the tip of the catheter in the right atrium. I then passed the special needle into the catheter and advanced it upward toward the right atrium, allowing the needle to rotate freely within the catheter as it was pushed toward the right atrium. The tip of the catheter and contained needle (positioned just inside the catheter tip) were then positioned against the bulge in the septum. Then, with considerable excitement and some trepidation, I pushed the needle forward and was elated to withdraw a highly oxygenated blood sample and to record a very high left atrial pressure with markedly abnormal pressure waves (fig. 12). Pressure was also recorded continuously as the transseptal needle was withdrawn across the septum from the left atrium into the right atrium (fig. 12). The patient lay quietly on the fluoroscopic table and reported no discomfort at any time during the procedure.

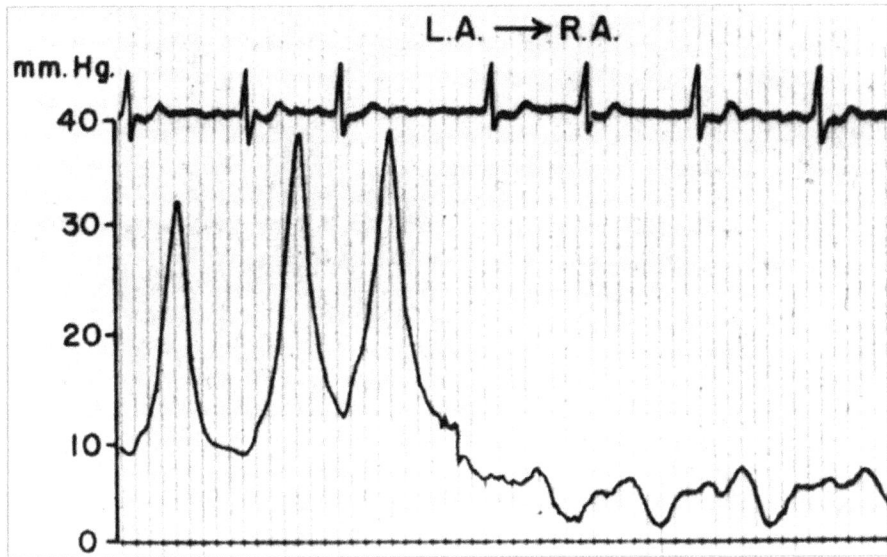

Figure 12. Left atrial pressure before and after
the transseptal needle was withdrawn
from the left atrium (L.A.) to the right atrium (R.A.)
in a patient with atrial fibrillation.
Am J Cardiol. 1959;3(5):655

In patients with a narrowed mitral valve (mitral stenosis), it was possible to pass a small plastic catheter through the needle after puncture of the atrial septum and to advance it into the left ventricle. Measurement of left atrial and left ventricular pressures and the cardiac output (by the indicator dilution method) allowed calculation of the severity of mitral valve narrowing in order to decide whether or not surgical treatment to open the valve was indicated.

A Useful Lesson for the Investigator About Sharing Preliminary Research

In 1958, I had reported at a meeting and published a short paper about the development of what I then named transseptal left heart catheterization, first in experimental animals[14] and then in humans.[15] Among those who expressed interest in the approach was a cardiologist who approached me, stating that his name was Dr. Cope, and he asked if he could observe me performing a transseptal catheterization in a patient in the NIH Cardiac Catheterization Laboratory. He said that he had not been successful in performing the procedure in dogs. I acceded to his request. Imagine my surprise, when soon after the publication of our paper concerning the first ten patients studied by the transseptal method at the NIH,[16] a "preliminary report" was published by C. Cope in a surgical journal concerning two patients on whom the transseptal method was performed without citing our work, of which he was obviously aware.

Subsequent Development of Transseptal Left Heart Catheterization

Studies in humans using transseptal left atrial puncture followed in 1959[17] and the new diagnostic method of transseptal left heart catheterization was reviewed in 1960.[18] My method was later modified in several laboratories by passing a larger catheter with a tapered tip over the transseptal needle into the left heart. This larger catheter allowed selective

---

14 Ross, "Catheterization of the left heart," 297–300.
15 J. Ross Jr., E. Braunwald, and A. G. Morrow, "Transseptal Left Atrial Puncture; New Technique for the Measurement of Left Atrial Pressure in Man," *American Journal of Cardiology* 3, no. 5 (1959): 653–655.
16 Ross, Braunwald, and Morrow, "Transseptal Left Atrial," 653–655.
17 Ross, Braunwald, and Morrow, "Transseptal Left Atrial," 653–655.
18 J. Ross Jr., E. Braunwald, and A. G. Morrow, "Transseptal left heart catheterization: a new diagnostic method," *Prog Cardiovasc Dis* 2 (1960): 315–318.

angiography of the left ventricle (LV), which is useful for studying the anatomy of that chamber and the mitral and aortic valves, as well as for assessing the degree of any mitral valve regurgitation. Importantly, it also allows for assessment of the function of the LV (which can be impaired in late stage disease), by calculating the ejection fraction of the LV (the stroke volume divided by the end-diastolic volume).

With the increasing use of selective coronary arteriography described above, it was found to be quite easy to manipulate a catheter backward through the aortic valve into the left ventricle. Therefore, so-called retrograde catheterization of the left ventricle largely replaced the transseptal method for routine diagnostic studies of the left ventricle, sometimes accompanied by measurement of the pulmonary artery wedge pressure to reflect left atrial pressure.

In recent years, however, transseptal left heart catheterization has reemerged as a useful tool for treating a number of cardiac conditions, including mitral stenosis. Mitral stenosis impedes blood flow from the left atrium to the left ventricle inducing elevated pressures in the left atrium and in the vessels draining into the left atrium from the lungs, causing excessive fluid accumulation in the lungs and shortness of breath. Mitral stenosis usually occurs as a consequence of the scarring of the valve leaflets caused by rheumatic fever. It remains a common debilitating disorder throughout much of the underdeveloped world, despite the fact that the control of rheumatic fever by prompt treatment of streptococcal infections, as well as the prophylactic use of antibiotics, has greatly reduced the frequency of rheumatic fever in the United States and in many other countries. Treatment of mitral stenosis usually involved cardiac surgery, which often was not available in less developed countries. However, in 1980, Inoue invented a catheter-tip balloon device that, when positioned in the mitral valve using the transseptal method, could be inflated to open the narrowed valve.[19] This procedure has been used as an effective way to avoid open-heart surgery and relieve symptoms due to mitral stenosis. The so-called balloon valvuloplasty is used when the anatomy of the diseased valve is favorable, particularly when fibrosis of the valve is not severe.

The transseptal method is now also widely applied for diagnosing and treating electrical disorders of the heart. Catheters are passed via the transseptal route into the left atrium and the left ventricle in order to map the location of abnormal electrical pathways, or the sites of origin of rhythm disturbances; these sites can then be ablated by a catheter, which can apply radio frequency energy to destroy very small regions of heart tissue.[20] Such treatment can be used to prevent intermittent, very rapid heart rhythms, or to block abnormal conduction of electrical impulses from one region of the heart to another.

It has been gratifying to witness these innovative applications to therapy of a method I developed as a diagnostic tool over forty years ago. Transseptal left heart catheterization has also become one of the standard tools for pacemaker implantations, aortic valvuloplasty, and the placement of devices for temporary support of the circulation.

---

19 K. Inoue, T. Owaki, T. Nakamura, F. Kitamura, and N. Miyamoto, "Clinical application of transvenous mitral commissurotomy by a new balloon catheter," *J Thorac Cardiovasc Surg* 87, no. 3 (1984): 394–402.

20 R. De Ponti, M. Zardini, C. Storti, M. Longobardi, and J. A. Salerno-Uriarte, "Trans-septal catheterization for radiofrequency catheter ablation of cardiac arrhythmias," *Eur Heart J* 19 (1998): 943–950.

CARDIAC CATHETERIZATION

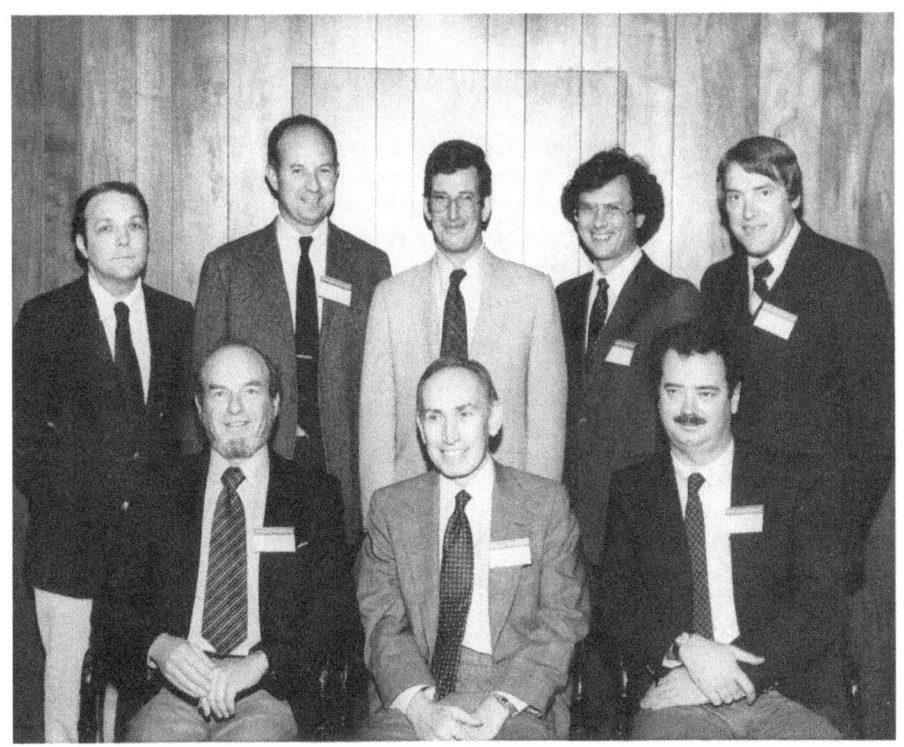

Figure 12.

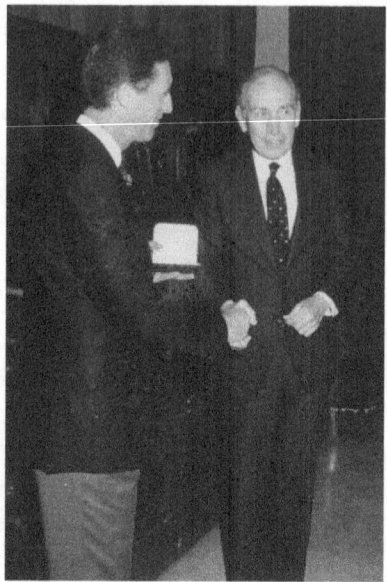

Figure 13.

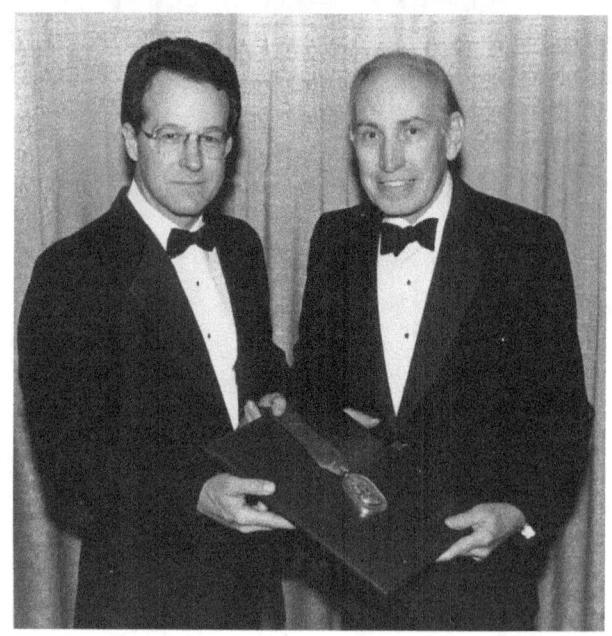

Figure 14.

CARDIAC CATHETERIZATION

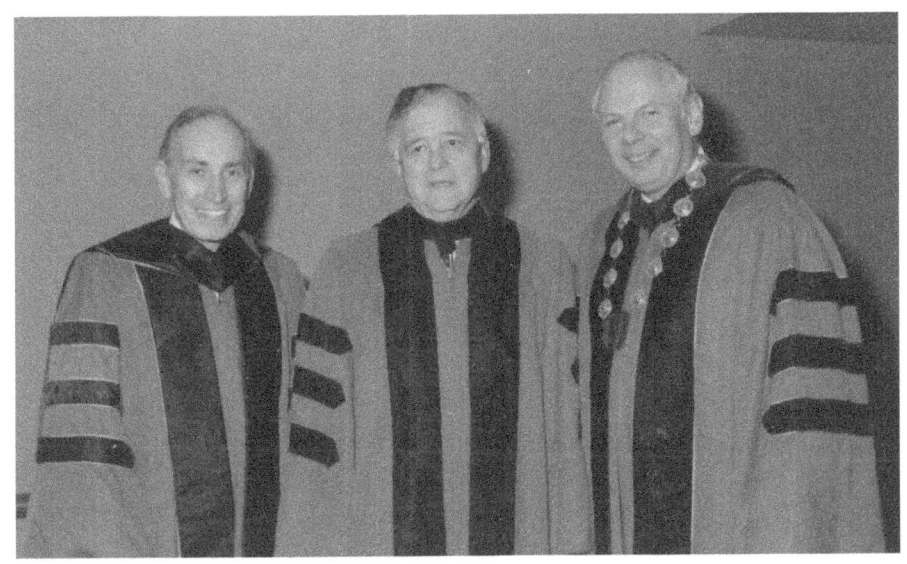

Figure 15.

CHAPTER 5
THE CONCEPT OF REPERFUSION AFTER CORONARY OCCLUSION

One research area of cardiology that I helped to initiate in the early 1970s concerns reopening a coronary artery after a period of coronary occlusion (reperfusion). Studies in animals in my experimental laboratory at the University of California San Diego demonstrated that it was possible to salvage large amounts of heart muscle by reopening a coronary artery (called "reperfusion"), even after three hours of coronary occlusion with substantial reduction in myocardial infarct size in the reperfused animals.[21] I proposed the potential for using this strategy

---

21 W. R. Ginks, H.D. Sybers, P. R. Maroko, J. W. Covell, B. E. Sobel, and J. Ross Jr., "Coronary Artery Reperfusion. II. Reduction of myocardial infarct size at 1 week after the coronary occlusion," *J Clin Invest* 51, no. 10 (1972): 2717–2723.

in humans after a coronary occlusion in an editorial in 1974.[22] By then, it had been well established that almost all coronary occlusions in patients with acute myocardial infarction were caused by a blood clot (thrombus) in a coronary artery.

In 1986, a large clinical trial in Italy of eleven thousand patients (the GISSI trial) clearly demonstrated that reperfusion by thrombolysis (dissolving the clot in the coronary artery) during a heart attack by giving the nonspecific enzyme streptokinase substantially lowered the death rate when administered during the first six hours after the onset of chest pain.[23] However, there was a small but significant incidence of bleeding in the gastrointestinal tract, the brain, or elsewhere with this treatment. This finding led to the development of an engineered drug, recombinant tissue plasminogen activator rtPA (alteplase), designed to affect only an established clot without causing bleeding elsewhere.

In 1990, a very large clinical trial (over 20,000 patients) compared alteplase with streptokinase;[24] this trial showed a slight further reduction of mortality with alteplase (about 1 percent) without substantially affecting the incidence of bleeding. Nevertheless, an advertising campaign in the United States resulted in widespread use of alteplase in this country, but not in many other parts of the world because the cost of rtPA was approximately tenfold higher than that of streptokinase. A group of academic scientists later showed that rtPA was twice as effective as streptokinase in opening coronary arteries within 90 minutes; the TIMI (Thrombolysis in Myocardial

---

22 J. Ross Jr., Editorial: "Early Revascularization After Coronary Occlusion. Circulation," 50, no. 6: 1061–1062.

23 Gruppo Italiano per lo Studio della Streptochinasi nel'Infarto Miocardico (GISSI), "Effectiveness of intravenous thrombolytic treatment in acute myocardial infarction," *Lancet* 1, no. 8478 (1986): 397–402

24 The International Study Group, "In-hospital mortality and clinical course of 20,891 patients with suspected acute myocardial infarction randomised between alteplase and streptokinase with or without heparin," *Lancet* 336 (1990): 71–5.

Infarction) group, founded by Dr. Eugene Braunwald, then went on to study a number of other strategies to produce rapid reperfusion of occluded coronary arteries by thrombolysis in patients within six hours of acute myocardial infarction.

In 1993, the GUSTO trial recruited over 40,000 patients to compare the effects of several thrombolytic strategies, in particular rtPA with streptokinase. It was theorized that the new agent would have a greater effect on lowering mortality and cause less bleeding than streptokinase. However, despite the large number of patients studied, the benefits were not impressive, mortality at thirty days being 6.3 percent with alteplase versus 7.4 percent for streptokinase.[25] This small difference was statistically significant, however, due to the large number of patients involved. With intense advertising, alteplase eventually became the drug of choice in the United States, despite a tenfold higher cost compared to streptokinase. The rest of the world largely saw the difference as minimal, and streptokinase remained the most common form of treatment outside of the United States. In the interim, different thrombolytic agents are being developed and research continues, stimulated by the TIMI group (Thrombolysis in Myocardial Infarction).[26]

---

25 "An international randomized trial comparing four thrombolytic strategies for acute myocardial infarction (GUSTO)," *NEJM* 329, no. 10 (1993): 673–682.
26 J. H. Chesebro, G. Knatterud, R. Roberts et al., "Thrombolysis in Myocardial Infarction (TIMI) Trial, Phase I: A comparison between intravenous tissue plasminogen activator and intravenous streptokinase," Clinical findings through hospital discharge. *Circulation* 76, no. 1 (1987): 142–154.

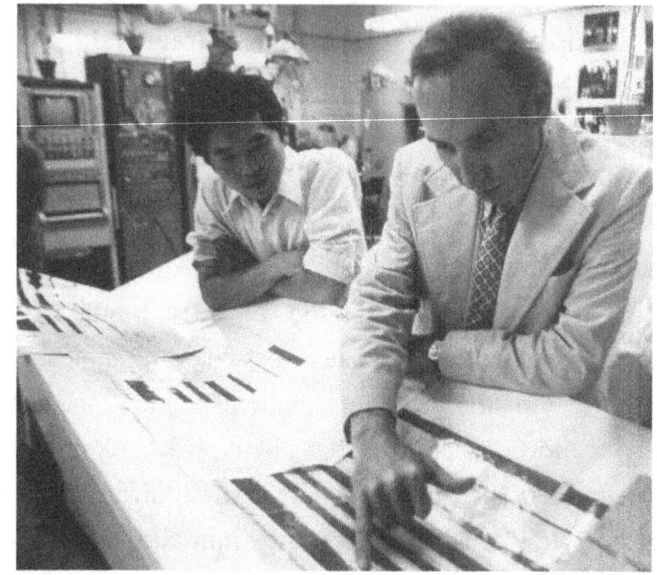

Figure 16.

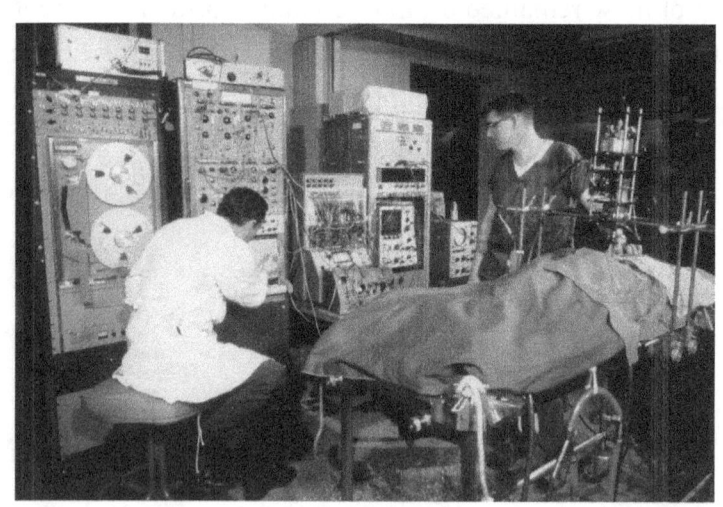

Figure 17.

THE CONCEPT OF REPERFUSION AFTER CORONARY OCCLUSION

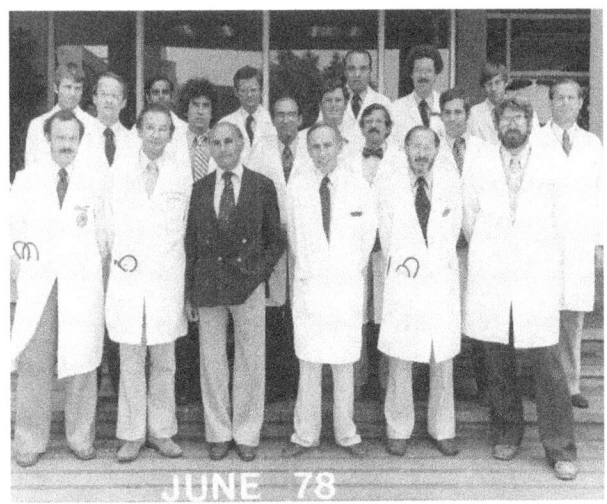

Figure 18.

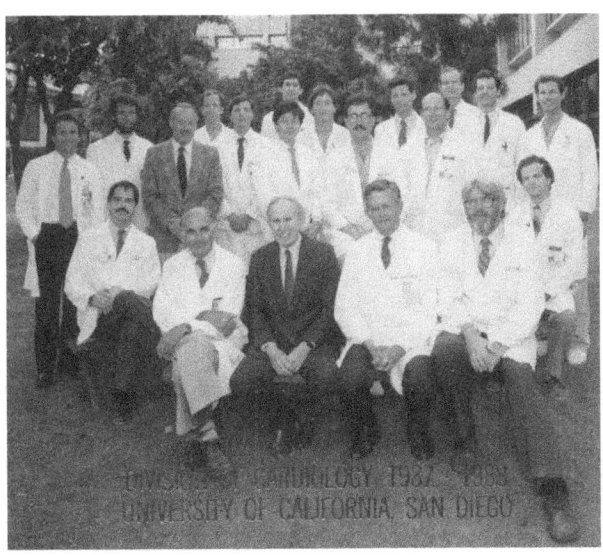

Figure 19.

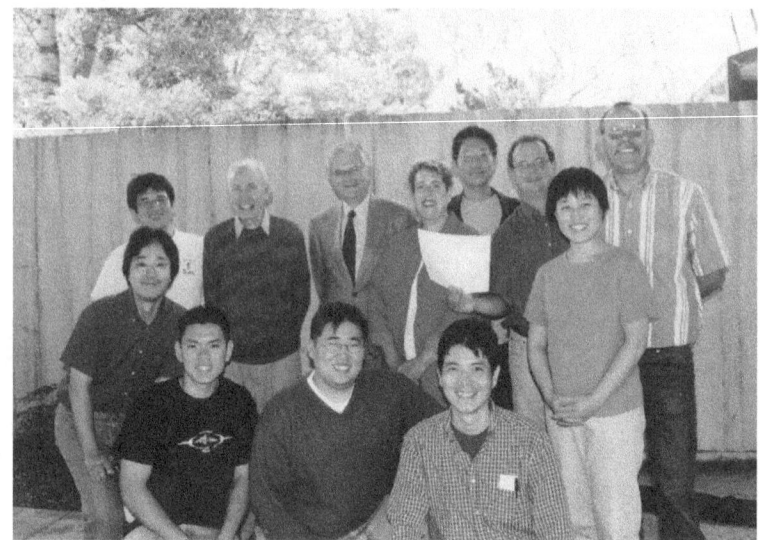

Figure 20.

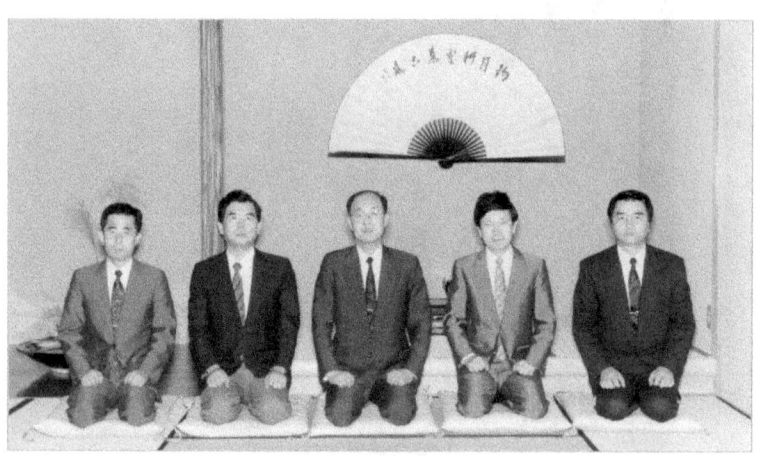

Figure 21.

CHAPTER 6
THE MOLECULAR/GENETIC REVOLUTION

Prior to the 1940s, most scientists believed that genetic information was transmitted by a protein. However, in the mid 1940s, a series of experiments published by Oswald Avery and his group documented that DNA (deoxyribonucleic acid), not a protein, was the "transforming factor" determining inheritance in bacteria.[27] Many have credited the origin of the revolution in molecular biology to the 1953 publication by James Watson and Francis Crick in the journal *Nature* of a model for the structure of DNA[28] for which they, together with Maurice Wilkins, received the Nobel Prize in Physiology and Medicine in 1962. It is interesting that Watson himself, in his remarkably frank 1968 book *The Double Helix*,[29] emphasized the key importance of x-ray crystallograph-

---

27 O. Avery, C. M. MacLeod, M. McCarty, "Studies on the chemical nature of the substance inducing transformation of pneumococcal types," *J Exp Med* 79, no. 2 (1944): 137–158.
28 J. D. Watson, F. Crick, "Molecular structure of nucleic acids: A Structure for Deoxyribose Nucleic Acid," *Nature* 171 (1953): 737–738.
29 James D. Watson, *The Double Helix: A Personal Account of the Discovery of the Structure of DNA* (New York: Kingsport Press Inc., 1968).

ic photos by Rosalind Franklin of one form of DNA in the development of their model (the so-called B form), which revealed the double helical structure of DNA. According to Watson, he glimpsed this photo when Wilkins took him into Franklin's laboratory.

Franklin published her findings and the DNA photo in a letter published in the same 1953 issue of *Nature*,[30] in which she indicated that her findings of DNA structure were compatible with the Watson/Crick model. In a separate letter in the same issue of *Nature*, Wilkins and coworkers cited their own x-ray diffraction studies in sperm heads and bacteriophage (both of which contain a high concentration of DNA), showing a helical structure of DNA in living creatures.[31]

It should be noted that although Watson was an American, he was working with Crick at the Cavendish Laboratory in Cambridge, England, while Wilkins and Franklin were at King's College in London, but their research efforts appear to have been more competitive than collaborative. Rosalind Franklin died in 1958 and received little recognition at the time, although much later Watson wrote a tribute to her in his 1968 book.[32] She could not be included in the 1962 Nobel Prize, since these are not awarded posthumously.

The DNA double helix, which forms the backbone of the DNA molecule, consists of two strands, each composed of alternating DNA and phosphate groups. Between these phosphate groups, pairs of purine and pyrimidine bases are attached in series. (fig. 22). An important component of the Watson/Crick model was the positioning of these sequential base pairs aligned within the DNA helix.

---

30 R. E. Franklin, R. G. Gosling, "Molecular Configuration in Sodium Thymonucleate," *Nature* 171 (1953): 740–741.
31 M. H. Wilkins, A. R. Stokes, and H. R. Wilson, "Molecular structure of deoxypentose nucleic acids," *Nature* 171, no. 4356 (1953): 738–740.
32 Watson, *The Double Helix*.

THE MOLECULAR/GENETIC REVOLUTION

Erwin Chargaff was said to be impressed by Oswald Avery's work on DNA, and reported an important insight: In DNA samples obtained from many different species, there was always a one to one ratio between the amount of purines (composed of adenine and guanine) and total pyrimidines (thymine plus cytosine).[33] Working with cardboard cutouts of the actual shape of these four bases, together with the double helix model that they had reproduced in wire, Watson and Crick, largely by trial and error, discovered that Chargaff was right. When adenine was paired with thymine, and guanine was paired with cytosine, the pair sizes were identical, and they fit precisely within the known dimensions of the double helix.[34] It was later shown that the sequence of these base pairs carries the genetic coding information, which is replicated during reproduction. Watson and Crick wrote in their 1953 letter to *Nature*: "We wish to suggest a structure for the salt of deoxyribose nucleic acid (DNA). This structure has novel features which are of considerable biological interest," the letter began, and at the end: "it has not escaped our notice that the specific pairing we have postulated immediately suggests a possible copying mechanism for the genetic material."

---

33 E. Vischer, E. Chargaff, "The separation and quantitative estimation of purines and pyrimidines in minute amounts," *J Biol Chem* 176, no. 2 (1948): 703–14

34 Wilkins, Stokes, and Wilson, "Molecular structure of deoxypentose nucleic acids," 738–740.

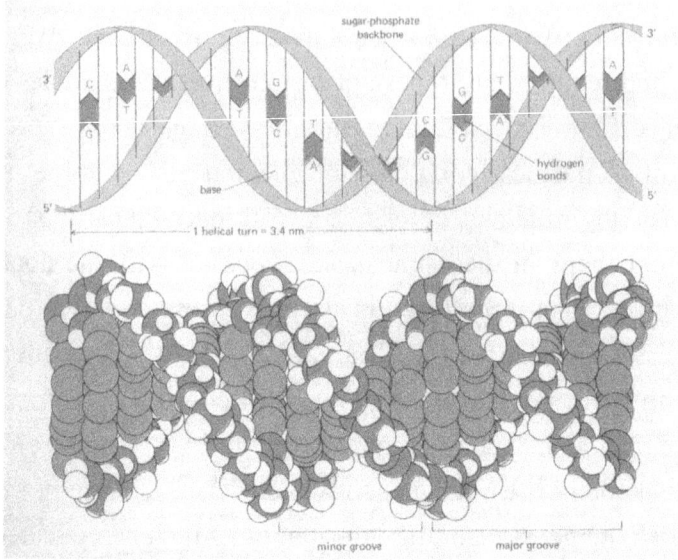

Figure 22. In a DNA molecule two antiparallel strands that are complementary in their nucleotide sequence are paired in a right-stranded double helix with about 10 nucleotide pairs per helical turn. A schematic representation (top) and a space-filling model (bottom) are illustrated here. "Copyright 1989 from *Molecular Biology of the Cell,* Second Edition by Alberts et al. Reproduced by permission of Garland Science/Taylor & Francis LLC."

What Is Molecular Medicine?

The early seminal work cited above provided the basis for much that has happened in the applications of molecular biology to human disease, including the mapping of the human genome, and the identification of specific gene defects as causes of some human diseases. This, in turn, stimulated the development of the field of molecular medicine, including the development of DNA transfer (gene therapy) and stem cell therapy.

Although full integration of these approaches into clinical treatment lies largely in the future, the process of such integration has begun. Several goals of molecular therapy can be identified, and examples of initial applications of molecular approaches to the treatment of human disease can be provided. In the future, the overriding theme of such treatments will likely be concerned with *targeting* specific therapies to identified disease mechanisms. By this I refer to the delivery of an agent (a gene, or a small molecule, a peptide, or an engineered drug) having relative specificity for a certain type of receptor molecule, if possible, one involved in the mechanism of a specific disease abnormality.

Research in cardiology was rather late to join the movement to molecular medicine, while molecular biological research in genetics, hematology, metabolism, and oncology (cancer) were realizing substantial advances. Perhaps this delay occurred in the cardiovascular area because of a series of rather spectacular breakthroughs in other disciplines that substantially improved the care and life expectancy of patients with heart disease.

Growth Factors and Inhibitors

Research is underway to identify small peptides that act to stimulate the proliferation of certain cell types, to, for example, stimulate specific cell types to grow in culture outside the body for later transplantation. Also, research is focused on developing inhibitors of specific growth factors that may be involved in certain diseases. An example of development in the latter area has provided a potential treatment for one form of loss of vision, macular degeneration. In older individuals this condition causes progressive loss of central vision in both eyes and is associated with tissue overgrowth and a variety of lesions of small blood vessels that supply the macular region of the retina. Leakage of blood and plasma from these vessels is associated with areas of degeneration and fibrosis in the retina. Efforts to treat this so-called exudative type of macular degeneration with photocoagulation or laser therapy have met with limited success. Physicians have experimentally used an inhibitor of a vascular growth factor, which was originally developed for the treatment of colorectal cancer (Avastin), for this condition. The inhibitor is injected in small doses directly into the eye, and initial reports indicate that it causes the damaged blood vessels to regress, thereby preventing leakage. A derivative drug (also developed by Genentech) is now in clinical trials. These agents may be the first to actually improve vision in this condition, in addition to slowing its progression.

Another example of a major advance in molecular research occurred in the 1980s, not in cardiology but in the field of metabolism, which later had a profound effect on the treatment of cardiovascular disease: the identification by Brown and Goldstein of the important enzyme in the liver that controls cholesterol synthesis (HMG-CoA reductase) and their development of an inhibitor of that enzyme,[35] for which they received the 1985 Nobel Prize in Physiology and Medicine. This inhibitor, called lovastatin, had an important effect on the development of coronary artery atherosclerosis by lowering the level of LDL cholesterol in the blood. Later generations of statin drugs are in widespread use for the prevention of atherosclerosis in blood vessels throughout the body; they are also used for slowing the progression of coronary artery atherosclerosis in patients with unstable disease, or those who have had a myocardial infarction, coronary bypass surgery, or coronary angioplasty.

---

35 T. F. Osborne, J. L. Goldstein, M. S. Brown MS, "5' End of HMG CoA Reductase Gene Contains Sequences Responsible for Cholesterol-Mediated Inhibition of Transcription," *Cell* 42, no.1 (1985): 203–12.

THE MOLECULAR/GENETIC REVOLUTION

A Molecular Treatment for Cancer

Conventional treatment for relatively advanced cancer involves the use of drugs that are highly toxic to cancer cells, but also affect normal cells and, therefore, cause severe side effects such as hair loss, nausea, vomiting, and weight loss. Not long ago, the FDA approved, in record time, a drug called Gleevec.[36] It was initially developed for a particular form of leukemia, the chronic myeloid type. Patients with this form of cancer have an abnormal chromosome, the Philadelphia chromosome, which leads to the production of an abnormal protein (a kinase), which promotes uncontrolled production of white blood cells. A scientist employed by a pharmaceutical company developed an agent designed to block this particular kinase, thereby inhibiting this signaling pathway and preventing production of the abnormal protein within the cancer cells.[37] Such cells require this activity, and when deprived of it, they die. Initial studies demonstrated that in over 90 percent of such patients, Gleevec produced a remission, which was often prolonged, allowing the number of white blood cells on the blood to return to normal. Side effects were mild to moderate, and the drug could be taken orally. Although long- term studies are currently underway, the drug has also been found useful for some other types of cancer.

Stem Cells, Embryonic and Other

There are several types of stem cells. The most primitive cell type found in mammals is the embryonic stem cell (ESI cell), which, under proper conditions, can develop into any cell types. Such cells

---

36 US Food and Drug Administration, Center for Drug Evaluation and Research. Gleevec NDA 21-335 approval letter February 27, 2001, from www.accessdata.fda.gov/drugsatfda_docs/appletter/2001/21335ltr.pdf

37 US Food and Drug Administration, Gleevec NDA 21-335 approval letter February 27, 2001.

are therefore said to be "pluripotent." During development of the normal embryo, such cells differentiate into the various tissues and organs of the body in a complex process under the control of multiple growth and differentiation factors. During this process, other forms of stem cells appear, which are further along in development; these are called progenitor cells. Such cells are no longer pluripotent but rather are already committed to develop in a certain direction. The latter cells can also be found in adult mammals, for example in bone marrow, skeletal muscle, and the central nervous system; also, they can be identified in human umbilical cord blood taken at the time of delivery. Once they are outside the body, specific molecular markers on progenitor cells allow them to be detected and sorted from other cells.

There has been some controversy in the United States on the potential uses of ES cells. Most often these cells are obtained from fertilized human ova (female human eggs) and stored for use during in vitro fertilization in fertilization clinics. Most of these eggs, if not used, are eventually discarded. When such fertilized eggs are grown in culture, the egg divides and continues to divide to produce what is called an embryoid body (a very early primitive embryo), which contains some cells that are already committed to early organ formation and other cells that are pluripotent. These human ES cells can be separated out using molecular markers. The National Academy of Sciences of the United States has issued guidelines for such procedures. However, ethical issues are raised by some groups, which equate the use of such primitive embryos with the killing of a human being.

Of course, such fertilized ova might be used for cloning an entire human, as has now been accomplished in sheep, cats, and dogs. Any attempt at such reproductive cloning of humans has been condemned by scientists and many others, as well as by the US government and most other countries. On the other hand, "therapeutic cloning" of human ES cells for the purpose of producing specific tissues or organs in order to replace diseased tissue or organs continues to be endorsed by many medical and basic scientists, and by the public in general. Such an application could be considered free of political, religious, and ethical issues. By culturing ES cells and adding differentiation and growth factors, specific cell types or tissues might be produced. This process could be made patient-specific by inserting an individual's DNA into the nucleus of a fertilized ovum. Although much research remains to be done in these areas, the successful production of genetically engineered patient-specific tissues would minimize the risk of rejection of transplanted tissue.

It was reported in the journal *Nature*[38] that human ES cells could be derived from single cells taken from very tiny embryos, comprised of only eight to ten cells, without appearing to harm the embryo. This approach might provide a source of human ES cells that could circumvent the objections of those who oppose destroying even primitive embryos in order to obtain ES cells, and perhaps remove much of the political cloud hampering research in these areas.

Applications of Stem Cell Therapy

Relatively differentiated forms of stem cells (progenitor cells) have been used in therapy for a number of years. For example, stem cells are present in the bone marrow obtained from a normal donor for a bone marrow transplantation procedure. These bone marrow cells

---

[38] I. Klimanskaya, Y. Chung, S. Becker, S. J. Lu, and R. Lanza, "Human embryonic stem cell lines derived from single blastomeres," *Nature* 444 (2006): 481–485.

(including bone marrow stem cells) have been matched using tissue typing procedures to a patient who has, for instance, an advanced form of leukemia or lymphoma in which conventional treatment is no longer effective. The patient is first treated with a heavy dose of radiation and/or chemotherapy to destroy all the cancer cells in the bone marrow and elsewhere. Of course, this will also destroy the patient's own bone marrow cells. Then, the donor's bone marrow cells are transplanted into the patient's bone marrow at a number of sites where, if the transplant is successful, the noncancerous stem cells will generate new cells that will differentiate into all of the normal blood cell types (red blood cells, white blood cells, and platelets). Donor matching is rarely precise, and drugs such as cyclosporin are given after transplantation to suppress any immune reactions to the transplant. Such treatment has prolonged many lives and in some instances resulted in the cure of certain types of cancer.[39]

Research is now underway on the use of other types of progenitor cells in addition to ES cells. For example, in early research, muscle stem cells separated from the skeletal muscle of a normal donor have been implanted for the treatment of muscular dystrophy.[40] Such cells have also been injected into the heart in patients who have suffered a heart attack followed by heart failure. These muscle progenitor cells may then develop into new cardiac muscle cells. Such studies are still in an early phase, and initial research in humans is inconclusive, although

---

39 A. Kessinger, J. O. Armitage, J. D. Landmark, D. M. Smith, and D. D. Weisenburger, "Autologous peripheral hematopoietic stem cell transplantation restores hematopoietic function following marrow ablative therapy," *Blood* 71, no. 3 (1988): 723–7.
40 M. Meregalli, A. Farini, D. Parolini, S. Maciotta, and Y. Torrente, "Stem Cell Therapies to Treat Muscular Dystrophy: progress to date," *BioDrugs* 24, no. 4 (2010): 237–47.

laboratory research in animals has demonstrated the feasibility of stem cell approaches for regenerating several types of tissue.[41]

Research is also ongoing on the use of stem cells for nerve regeneration. A group of investigators has described a complex process involving the use of rat ES cells to treat virus-induced paralysis of the hind limbs.[42] In these rats, restoration of functional connections between nerve fibers and muscle cells was accomplished by transplanting ES cells into damaged areas and at the same time injecting a nerve growth factor into the nerve where it exits from the spinal cord. Other factors are also administered to inhibit the deleterious effects of myelin, which surrounds the normal nerve fibers and inhibits the growth of new nerve fibers. These experiments showing successful treatment of paralysis in rats offer promise for eventual application in humans.

Gene Therapy

Delivery of genes is another area in which promising research is underway. An investigation in our laboratory at UCSD provides an example of how a gene can be successfully transferred to the heart, and the approach may find applications in humans with certain forms of heart disease. In 25 to 30 percent of human subjects with dilated cardiomyopathy, the cause of heart disease is genetic in origin and, while many different genes are involved, the end result is a heart with abnormally thin walls due to loss of muscle cells leading to enlargement

---

[41] W. E. Wang, X. Chen, S. R. Houser, and C. Zeng, "Potential of cardiac stem/progenitor cells and induced pluripotent stem cells for cardiac repair in ischaemic heart disease," *Clin Sci (Lond)* 125, no. 7 (2013): 319–27.

[42] D. M. Deshpande, Y.S. Kim, T. Martinez et al., "Recovery from Paralysis in Adult Rats Using Embryonic Stem Cells," *Ann Neurol* 60 (2006): 32–44.

of the heart chambers (dilation), reduced heart function, and eventual heart failure.

A form of genetic dilated cardiomyopathy in the hamster has been recognized for many years, and a company now breeds such animals for use in research. Recently, researchers in Italy and Japan have identified the gene mutation responsible for this condition in the hamster (the same gene is also involved in rare cases of cardiomyopathy in humans). The gene codes for a key protein, which is a component of the structural connection between the inside and the outside of the cardiac muscle cells (the so-called dystrophin-dystroglycan complex), and this protein, delta sarcoglycan, is absent in the cardiomyopathic hamster heart.[43]

At UCSD, we undertook a feasibility study in these hamsters to determine if the missing gene could be replaced. First, we developed a method involving gene delivery directly into the aorta. The method could be used to insert a gene into the hearts of living hamsters, leading to high efficiency expression in about 65 percent of the muscle cells of the main pumping chamber, the left ventricle. Then we attached the missing delta sarcoglycan gene to a virus that had been engineered so that it could not reproduce but could nevertheless carry the gene into the heart muscle cells.[44] Then this viral-gene vector was infused through the coronary arteries to reach the heart muscle. We were able to show that the gene entered the muscle cells and that the missing protein was produced, so that three weeks later we could stain it in the cell membranes of 70 percent of the cells in the left ventricle. The result was substantial

---

[43] M. Hoshijima, T. Hayashi, Y. E. Jeon, Z. Fu, Y. Gu, N. D. Dalton, M. H. Ellisman, X. Xiao, F. L. Powell, and J. Ross Jr., "Delta-sarcoglycan Gene Therapy Halts Progression of Cardiac Dysfunction, Improves Respiratory Failure, and Prolongs Life in Myopathic Hamsters," *Circ Heart Fail* 4, no. 1 (2011):89–97.

[44] Hoshijima et. al., "Delta-sarcoglycan Gene Therapy," 89–97.

improvement in the structure and function of the damaged heart (fig. 23 and 24). In the future it may become feasible to insert a normal gene into the hearts of patients with a specific genetic mutation that causes cardiomyopathy.

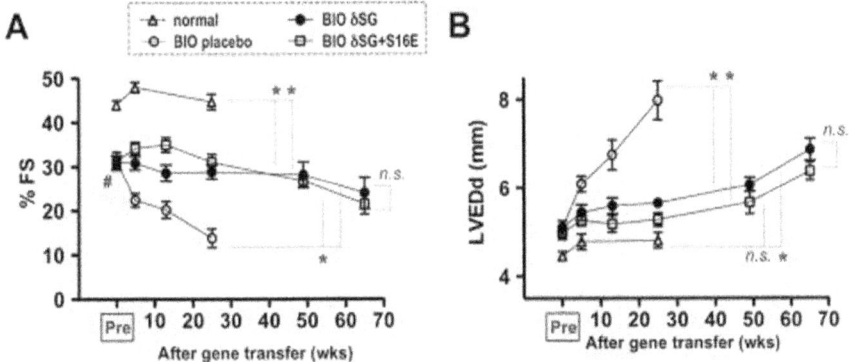

Figure 23. (A) Preservation of % fractional shortening (%FS) by delta-sarcoglycan treatment.
(B) Prevention of LV dilation, left ventricular end-diastolic dimension (LVEDd) with treatment.
Circ Heart Fail. 2011;4(1):89–97.

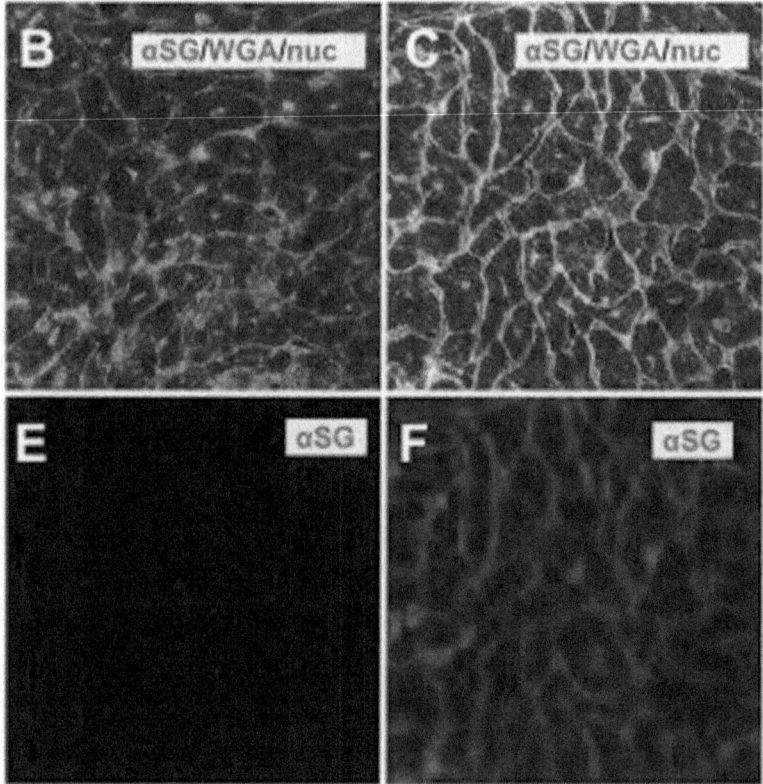

Figure 24. Reconstitution of the DGC by δSG GT in cardiomyocytes. LV tissues were collected from BIO14.6 hamsters after 28 weeks of treatment with δSG/AAV9 alone. The effect of δSG/AAV9 treatment (C and F) in BIO14.6 hamsters was referenced to placebo treatment (B and E). E and F, αSG staining (red) alone. B and C, combination of αSG staining (red) with membrane staining with WGA (green), which stains both the peripheral sarcolemma and T system, and nuclear staining (nuc, blue) with DAPI. Circ Heart Fail. 2011;4(1):89–97.

Efforts are now underway in several centers to develop the techniques necessary to treat human heart failure (after a heart attack or other conditions, such as longstanding hypertension). In end-stage human heart failure, there is usually a defect in the uptake and release of calcium during each heart contraction. In experimental animals, delivery of a gene which codes for the expression of a specific protein, sarco/endoplastmic reticulum (SERCA) Ca2+ ATPase, responsible for the uptake and release of calcium within the muscle cells, leads to improved heart function. A clinical trial of this approach to treatment is currently planned in patients with heart failure.

There is also the possibility of delivering other genes that can produce proteins that may be therapeutic for a variety of other disease conditions in different organs, such as delivery of a gene to the lungs for the treatment of cystic fibrosis.

A Combined Treatment Approach

A final example of the potential for molecular medicine is provided by a clinical application of both gene therapy and stem cell therapy to treat a human disease. This study, reported in 2002 by French scientists, described the first successful long term cure of a rare inherited disease called SCID (severe combined immunodeficiency disease)[45] in which fatal infections occur during the first year of life if the baby is left untreated. Several years ago SCID became known as "bubble boy disease," after a child who was maintained under relatively sterile conditions within a large plastic bubble in order to avoid infections. This approach proved successful for twelve years, but the child finally died in 1984. The genetic mutation in this disorder is sex-linked, so it occurs only in males, and the mutation results in a missing protein necessary for the production of certain types of white blood cells essential for fighting infections. After obtaining appropriate approvals from French government agencies and

---

45 L. M. Muul, L. M. Tuschong, S. L. Soenen, G. J. Jagadeesh, W. J. Ramsey, Z. Long, C. S. Carter, E. K. Garabedian, M. Alleyne, M. Brown, W. Bernstein, S. H. Schurman, T. A. Fleisher, S. F. Leitman, C. E. Dunbar, R. M. Blaese, and F.Candotti, "Persistence and expression of the adenosine deaminase gene for 12 years and immune reaction to gene transfer components: long-term results of the first clinical gene therapy trial," *Blood* 107, no. 7 (2003): 2563–9.

the local ethics committee, along with informed consent from the parents, babies with SCID between the ages of one and eleven months were enrolled in the study.[46] Samples of bone marrow were then obtained in which stem cells were identified, isolated, and cultured outside the body.

These isolated cultured stem cells then underwent gene therapy using a vector containing a nonreplicating virus attached to the key portion of the DNA in the missing gene; the cells subsequently produced the missing protein using the inserted DNA, and they were maintained in culture, where they continued to divide until millions of stem cells were available for each patient. These cells were then given to populate the bone marrows of these patients, and because the cells were autologous (each child received its own modified stem cells), no rejection response to the administered cells was observed. After follow-up periods as long as three and one-half years, four of the five children had normal bone marrow function, normal circulating white blood cells, and were free of disease.[47]

It seems unlikely that gene or stem cell treatment will become commonplace in clinical medicine in the near future; however, preclinical research in animals has proven the feasibility and great potential of molecular treatments, and such research offers hope for patients with diseases for which conventional treatments are not effective.

---

46 R. M. Blaese, K. W. Culver, A. D. Miller et al., "T Lymphocyte-Directed Gene Therapy for ADA SCID: Initial Trial Results After 4 Years," *Science* 270, no. 5235 (1995):475–480.

47 Blaese, Culver, Miller et al., "T Lymphocyte-Directed Gene Therapy," 475–480.

CHAPTER 7
ON ASSESSING MEDICAL RESEARCH

For over thirty-five years as a professor of medicine and cardiology at the University of California San Diego School of Medicine, I lectured to medical students on cardiovascular physiology and heart disease and taught students in the clinics and on the medical wards of our teaching hospital. I also consulted in the hospital, saw outpatients, and carried out laboratory and clinical research programs. One of my most rewarding teaching experiences was as an annual lecturer to a large class of undergraduate junior and senior university students at UCSD, many of whom were planning to apply to medical school or for other training in health care delivery. The course, entitled "The Anthropology of Medicine,"[48] was designed and conducted by my wife and fellow professor at the UCSD School of Medicine, anthropologist Lola Romanucci. I gave a lecture in the course to this nonmedical audience in which I summarized my own experiences and views

---

48 L. RomanucciRoss and D. Moerman, *The Anthropology of Medicine: From Culture to Method* (Abbey Publishing, 1985).

on how audience members should consider information about medical research findings from various sources, and how they should take responsibility for their own health by keeping well informed while maintaining an inquiring yet skeptical attitude.

Researchers and practicing physicians are inundated with enticing results from trials of new medications. There was a time not so long ago when the "ethical pharmaceutical companies" (as they were then called) advertised only to physicians, nurses, and other health professionals. Not any longer. In recent years the industry has spent huge sums for direct advertising to the public, as well as for lobbying Congress and the administration for favorable legislation and rulings (such as preventing the sale in the United States of lower cost drugs from Canada). These practices have added greatly to the rapidly escalating cost of medications. Today, the major companies (so-called big pharma) claim that these high prices are due to the expense of developing new products. Although the latter process is costly and can be prolonged, it is clear that full-page newspaper ads and frequent television spots have been a highly effective marketing strategy, reflected in drug sales and huge company profits, while prices for drugs continue to increase. Of course, an informed public might be a desirable side effect of such advertising, but it is not clear how useful ads are which often end with "ask your doctor if drug X is right for you."

In addition to advertising, what other sources for information about drugs (and other medical matters) are available to consumers and would-be patients? The original sources are reports of scientific research in patients published in scientific journals. These publications may be summarized with reasonable accuracy in some newspapers and magazine articles; however, it is quite common to see press releases, often an announcement prior to publication, sometimes by a biotech company, concerning highly promising results with a new agent. Such announcements commonly exaggerate the importance of the findings (often serving to boost the price of the company's stock).

Types of Research

Research may be laboratory based (not in human subjects), including applied research in animal models of disease, epidemiological research in humans, or a clinical trial involving a medication or a procedure. Examples of basic research are discoveries of biochemical pathways, or genetic mutations in cells that may later lead to specific drugs. Examples of applied laboratory research might include testing the effects in animals of coronary artery occlusion, followed by directly reopening the artery (reperfusion), or by inducing a blood clot in the coronary artery and then infusing a thrombolytic (clot dissolving) drug. Clinical research can include a small observational trial of a new drug, or a large-scale clinical trial designed to study the effects of a new drug on mortality, symptoms, and adverse effects in a given disease compared to conventional treatment.

Reading about such research can include the original journal article, but for the nonprofessional the most likely source is often a newspaper or magazine summary, or a story on television. In any case, it is valuable to have some understanding about what constitutes reliable laboratory research, types of epidemiological research, and the ingredients of a valid clinical trial.

Laboratory Research

Laboratory research requires a phenomenon or theory that can be tested, an accurate and reproducible method to measure the response (be it molecular, biochemical, or physiological), a sufficient number of observations to assure that the observed responses are not due to chance variations (usually requiring statistical testing), and an interpretation of the findings by the authors (sometimes the weakest part of the presentation). Such interpretation may reflect bias toward a favorable outcome, and should be accepted with caution only after learning the details of the study. The importance of interpretations of research can be highlighted in the courtroom, where expert witnesses for opposing sides (who may be physicians, PhDs, and/or experts in various disciplines) may give entirely opposite conclusions about the value of a published study. So-called junk science is a popular term for some of these discussions.

Epidemiological Research

Epidemiological research can be extremely valuable; common types of epidemiological research are cross-sectional studies and longitudinal studies. An example of the former are called case control studies, in which, at a given point in time, two sizeable populations are matched in as many features as possible (gender, occupation, socio-economic level, region of the country, diet, and environmental factors, etc.), except for one factor. When, for example, that factor was smoking and studies compared those who smoked to those who did not smoke, study after study showed a higher risk of lung cancer in the smoking group. These case control studies stimulated basic research on the carcinogenic effects of components of tobacco smoke, which led to campaigns against smoking and the later discovery that smoking also increases the risk of heart attack.

Another example of cross-sectional research is the famous Seven Countries Study,[49] in which dietary habits of populations in differ-

---

[49] A. Trichopoulou, T. Costacou, C. Bamia, and D. Trichopoulos, "Adherence to a Mediterranean Diet and Survival in a Greek Population," *N Engl J Med* 348, no. 26 (2003): 2599–608.

ent countries were examined in detail. One important finding was that the "Mediterranean diet," ingested by Italian fishermen, was associated with a low risk of heart attack in contrast to the standard European or American diet, high in fat, meats, and dairy products. The Mediterranean diet featured not only fish but also liberal use of olive oil (a mono-unsaturated oil, now known to be heart-healthy), low intake of red meat and fat, and liberal ingestion of pasta, tomatoes, and other vegetables. This study was instrumental in focusing attention to the importance of a healthy diet and its relation to cholesterol in the blood, which has continued to grow in interest ever since.

One problem with this type of study is that factors not accounted for can influence findings. Factors such as environmental agents that cannot be measured or environmental and cultural factors that play a large but unknown role in one group but not the other, may not be considered by the investigators. Thus, it is always prudent to watch for other confirmatory studies of different design from different locations or countries.

What about longitudinal epidemiological studies? One investigation of this type is the Framingham Study, funded by the National Institutes of Health.[50] Beginning over forty years ago in the small Massachusetts town of Framingham (population about five thousand), this study has continued to this day. At the outset, a number of factors including weight, age, gender, health history, blood pressure, the electrocardiogram, serum cholesterol, smoking history, family history, amount and type of exercise, and other variables were recorded. All these individuals were examined periodically over the years for cardiovascular and other

---

50 W. B. Kannel, T. R. Dawber, A. Kagan, N. Revotskie, and J. Stokes, "Factors of Risk in the Development of Coronary Heart Disease-Six-Year Follow-up Experience The Framingham Study," *Ann Intern Med* 55, no. 1 (1961): 33–50.

significant medical events. The Framingham Study clearly established the risk factors for cardiac events, including fatal and nonfatal heart attacks. Among these risk factors are what I call "the big three," because they can be modified: elevated blood pressure (typically at least 140/90), elevated serum cholesterol, and a history of sustained smoking. Other less powerful risk factors were found, and many of these can also be modified; they include physical inactivity, obesity, diabetes, stress, and an emerging risk factor, the blood level of C–reactive protein, a marker of inflammation, which is now considered important in the development of atherosclerotic plaques in blood vessels.

There are two other major risk factors that cannot be altered: genetic history and gender. A family history of premature heart attack in a close relative is highly predictive, and men tend to have heart attacks about ten years earlier than women.

Research on New Medications and Procedures

These appear almost daily in the public media. Many such studies are conducted on small numbers of patients in which the patients are followed for relatively short periods; these can be called "observational studies." Such research can be highly useful in initial testing for safety and efficacy of a new drug. An example is provided by the early studies on medications for lowering blood pressure in patients with hypertension (high blood pressure). Some of the initial medications used in the 1950s and 1960s, such as reserpine, or drugs that block the autonomic nervous system, were shown to be moderately effective and relatively safe, but they often had significant side effects. Later studies established that more powerful and safer agents, such as angiotensin converting enzyme inhibitors, calcium channel blockers, and beta-adrenergic blocking drugs, had greater effectiveness in lowering blood pressure. However, the initial observational studies did not have a large enough population or long enough duration of follow-up to allow reliable conclusions about the consequences of sustained hypertension (in particular stroke and premature heart attack). Could these events, which are often fatal, be prevented by treatment with such medications?

Observational trials on treating hypertension were successful in showing major reductions in the incidence of stroke and stroke mortality in treated patients. Hypertension is known as the silent killer (because individuals can have significantly elevated blood pressure for many years without any symptoms), and many individuals with undiagnosed hypertension remain untreated. In the United States and Japan, major public education campaigns were undertaken along with hypertension detection and treatment programs. As a result, by the 1990s there were reductions of about 70 percent in the incidence of fatal stroke.[51] Later, a protective effect of hypertension treatment on heart attack (myocardial infarction) was also demonstrated.

The Clinical Trial

To answer many questions, the large-scale clinical trial, usually referring to a randomized clinical trial, has evolved in recent years into a formal and highly structured research tool. These trials might be sponsored by a pharmaceutical company (in which case, absence of conflict of interest must be assured), by government institutions in the United States or abroad, or in recent years, by combined sponsorships. Such studies have become numerous in all fields of medicine, although I will use examples

---

51 H. Iso, T. Shimamoto, Y. Naito et al., "Effects of a Long-term Hypertension Control Program on Stroke Incidence and Prevalence in a Rural Community in Northeastern Japan," *Stroke* 29 (1998): 1510–1518.

from the cardiovascular field. Features of such trials include (or should) include:
1. A sufficient number of patients in treated and untreated (control) groups for which expected events, such as fatal and nonfatal stroke, will occur at a relatively well known frequency in the untreated patients and at a lower frequency in the treated patients. To be proven statistically, this often requires that thousands of patients in each group are followed for several years.
2. The patients should be assigned in a randomized manner to a treatment pill (medication) or a placebo pill (sugar) by physicians who are "blinded," or unaware of which type of pill they administer (the patients are similarly blinded and unaware of which type of pill they receive). The purpose of blinding is to eliminate physician bias, which might favor assignment to active treatment of a patient with more severe disease. Blinding of patients is also done to eliminate phenomena that can occur when a patient knows that he or she is on active treatment; it is recognized that patients who know they are on treatment tend to report fewer symptoms than those who are not aware, and patients may exaggerate symptoms if on placebo.
3. Appointment of a data monitoring board, which periodically reviews the data as the trial progresses and can recommend ending the trial early if the results indicate either overwhelming benefit of the drug, or a clear increase on adverse effects in the drug-treated group.
4. An independent policy board, which approves the original design of the trial, decides whether or not to continue the trial to its scheduled end, oversees the statistical analyses, and works

with the trial investigators from many different centers and/or countries in preparing the results for publication.
5. The trial should meet ethical standards, an important part of which concerns the control group. In many early trials, the control group was untreated (placebo). However, as treatments became available and proved to be beneficial, it became unethical to deprive the control group of such medications, and today both the control and treatment groups receive conventional treatment with one or more medications, and comparison is made with the addition of the new medication only in the treatment group.

A historical example of an unethical study was performed in Tuskegee, Alabama, beginning in 1930 and spanning a number of years.[52] Conducted by a United Sates government research group, it was a longitudinal study of the late effects of syphilis in a population of black males designed to characterize and define late complications. The study was started before there was a genuinely effective treatment for syphilis, but when penicillin became available the study was continued for a number of years without using this effective, curative form of treatment. Needless to say, many individuals in the study developed late complications of syphilis, which could and should have been avoided. Depriving patients in any clinical study of treatment known to be efficacious is clearly not only unethical, but can have unconscionable and tragic consequences both for the patient and those with whom the patient is intimate, as it did in Tuskegee.

Several years ago, safeguards in clinical trial design were implemented after the publication of some egregiously mismanaged trials, usually performed by a sponsoring company, that failed to protect

---

[52] "Tuskegee Study - Timeline" NCHHSTP. CDC. 2008-06-25. Retrieved 2008-12-04.

against bias and conflict of interest, and thereby raised serious doubt about reported results.

In presenting types of medical research to our class of university students, I also discussed the so-called mega-trials, which involve thousands of patients. This type of trial is typically used to detect relatively uncommon events, so that the number of events in the control (untreated) group is sufficiently large that an adequate statistical comparison can be made for identifying a reduction of deaths, or adverse effects, in the treatment group. Perhaps the first mega-trial in the cardiovascular area was conducted in Italy; the GISSI trial (Groupo Italiano for the Study of Streptokinase in Infarction), involved 11,000 patients.[53] A long-held view asserted that a heart attack is caused by formation of a blood clot (thrombus) in one of the coronary arteries that supplies the heart with oxygenated blood, an event called a coronary occlusion (or "a coronary"), which leads to a myocardial infarction (death of region of heart tissue in the left ventricle supplied by that artery). A series of small studies conducted over a number of years, using intravenous injection of an enzyme (a thrombolytic agent) that can dissolve a thrombus, gave results that were variable and inconclusive. At about that time, coronary angiography was performed in a number of patients early after the onset of a heart attack allowing visualization of the obstructing clot and proving the above-mentioned theory of coronary occlusion. The GISSI trial randomized patients to placebo or to streptokinase (a thrombolytic, i.e., clot-dissolving agent) within six hours of onset of a myocardial infarction. The study demonstrated a 50 percent reduction in mortality with treatment within one hour of onset of chest pain, a 25 percent reduction within three hours, and a smaller

---

53 "Effectiveness of intravenous thrombolytic treatment in acute myocardial infarction. Gruppo Italiano per lo Studio della Streptochinasi nell'Infarto Miocardico (GISSI)," *Lancet* 1, no. 8447 (1986): 397–402.

but still significant reduction within six hours. This study, published in 1986, revolutionized the treatment of heart attacks and stimulated the pharmaceutical industry to produce new and better thrombolytic agents.

As valuable as clinical trials have been and continue to be, it is important to know that most of them are not of an appropriate size and duration to detect uncommon complications. Nevertheless, the US Food and Drug Administration (FDA) relies on them to decide whether or not to approve (release) a product for use by physicians for a particular indication. It should be noted that once a drug is released by the FDA, it may be used by physicians for other (nonapproved) purposes, for which it may not have been proven to be safe and effective, and it is only with very widespread use (millions rather than thousands of doses of a drug) that uncommon or rare, perhaps serious, adverse effects begin to be detected. One factor in the haste to get new drugs to market is the desire of patients and doctors to have better treatments available, but another, sometimes decisive, factor is pressure from the pharmaceutical industry on the FDA for faster and faster reviews. In releasing a product based on relatively small trials, the FDA is essentially relying on post-release information about uncommon adverse reactions to a drug. Post-trial complications are supposed to be carefully recorded by the company that makes the drug and reported to the FDA, but reporting by patients and physicians to the company is voluntary. From my own perspective, informed by my reporting of side effects to companies and my attempts to obtain information about post-trial complications, it is apparent that companies have little incentive to systematically gather and release such information. Thus, a patient may experience an adverse reaction, and it may never come to light. In addition, the FDA has often been slow to request withdrawal of a new drug, even when complaints become numerous. A recent case in point is a drug that was used in the treatment of diabetes but that caused liver damage in many patients and over eighty deaths before it was finally recalled. This problem has also been recently demonstrated with the widely advertised pain medications Vioxx and Celebrex (both COX-2 prostaglandin inhibitors), which, after release, were discovered to pose a small but significantly increased risk of heart attack.[54]

It is highly desirable that an individual become knowledgeable and involved in his or her own health, including the selection of treatment options in case of illness. A good way to begin to become knowledgeable (and careful) is to read the package insert for any prescribed medication. This sheet is sometimes included with the medication, but it is always available from the pharmacist upon request. The insert summarizes the results of relevant clinical trials of the drug, the percentage of patients who obtain effective control of symptoms, and the type and percentage of side effects. It also states the approved indications for use. This information should be discussed with a physician, and together the patient and physician should decide whether the potential risks are worth the expected benefits. But one should remember that the reported complications are only those from the published trials (unless the FDA has mandated a supplement describing additional post-trial complications), and such complications may be expected with any new drug.

The advertising fanfare that accompanies the release of a new drug often leads patients to request it from their doctor, and it has been reported that physicians are more likely to prescribe an advertised drug when it is specifically requested by a patient. Of course, it is important to remember that there are many drugs on the market with long established

---

[54] D. Mukherjee, S. E. Nissen, and E. J. Topol, "Risk of Cardiovascular Events Associated With Selective COX-2 Inhibitors," *JAMA* 286, no. 8 (2001): 954–9.

safety and efficacy records. These are often quite inexpensive, since US patents expire after twenty years, and generic drugs (which are exact replicas of the original) often become available. Therefore, it seems advisable to use one of these older products initially, if feasible, and to wait a year or two before taking a newly released one.

CHAPTER 8
INTERNATIONAL COLLABORATIONS

In 1982, Professor Dirk Brusaert, from Antwerp, Belgium, spent several weeks in La Jolla at the UCSD School of Medicine visiting with me and with my laboratory group, as well as with selected other faculty members. In 1983, I visited with Dr. Bruseart in Antwerp, and we planned a series of international scientific conferences. In 1987, Professor Chuichi Kawai and Dr. Shigetake Sasayama added Kyoto, Japan as a host site. Between 1984 and 2010 there were thirteen Antwerp/La Jolla/Kyoto conferences. In 2010, Dr. Gianluigi Condorelli added Italy to the rotation with subsequent meetings in Rome and on the island of Capri.

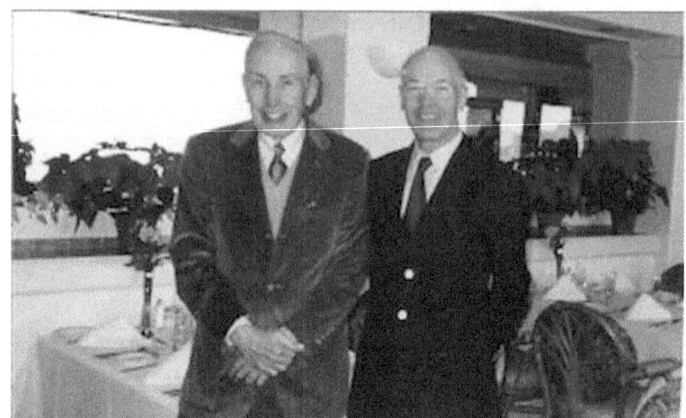

Figure 25.

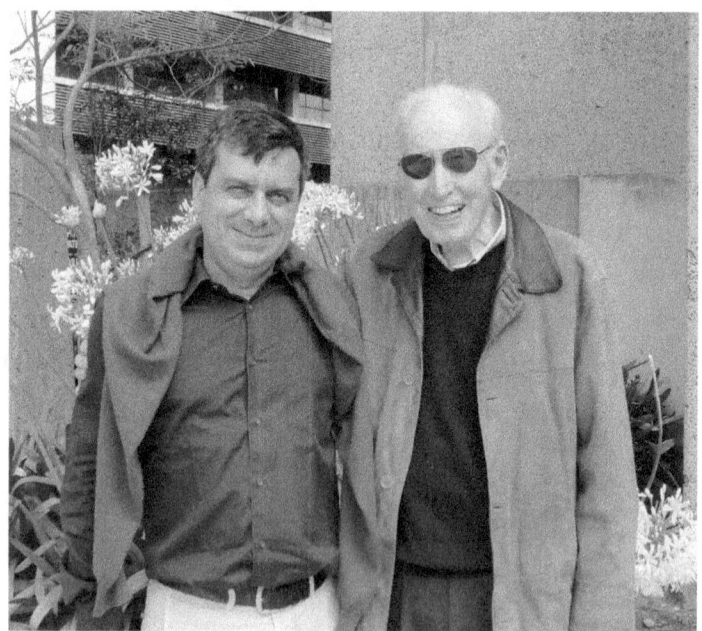

Figure 26.